Managing Segmental Renal Diseases

Salvatore Rocca Rossetti

Managing Segmental Renal Diseases

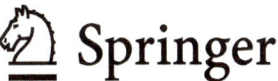 Springer

Salvatore Rocca Rossetti
Urology Department
University of Turin
Turin
Italy

ISBN 978-3-319-49720-4   ISBN 978-3-319-49721-1   (eBook)
DOI 10.1007/978-3-319-49721-1

Library of Congress Control Number: 2017955681

Printed on acid-free paper

This Springer imprint is published by Springer Nature
The registered company is Springer International Publishing AG
The registered company address is: Gewerbestrasse 11, 6330 Cham, Switzerland

Preface

Segmental renal diseases or pathologies are those occurring in a segment of an organ. A segment of the kidney, like those in the lung or liver, is not just any portion of the organ but a precise embryological and anatomically autonomous structural district with an equally autonomous function. Some diseases affect the kidney, temporarily, in a segment, respecting the rest of the organ; at this stage the pathology is segmental and if its treatment is surgical, the operation consists of a segmentectomy—that is, precise excision of the segment—leaving the rest of the kidney unscathed.

Study of the development of the kidney (embryology, organogenesis, and final constitution) has made it possible to establish a way to locate, reach, and remove each renal segment, i.e., renal lobe.

Segmental renal diseases and pathologies are not frequent, in fact they are rather rarer than those that are diffuse in the parenchyma or located in peripheral or nonsegmental areas of the kidney. Consequently, kidney segmentectomies (lobectomies) are indicated less frequently than other types of conservative surgery.

From a surgical point of view there is an essential difference in the aggressiveness of the technique in the kidney: endorenal in segmentectomies and extrarenal in tumorectomies, partial nephrectomies, and renal resections. Renal segmentectomies require a hilum–sinus approach; they are a typical kind of endorenal surgery.

The content of this book focuses on the peculiar character-istics of segmental renal diseases and pathologies, and anatomo-surgical aspects of endorenal surgery for specific segment removal in the kidney.

Turin, Italy   Salvatore Rocca Rossetti

Acknowledgments

The author would like to thank his colleagues and friends who agreed to contribute to this work with their opinions, comments, or suggestions: Dr. C. Boccafoschi, Head of Urological Private Department at Alessandria Clinic (Alessandria), Italy; Dr. A. Dezan, Head of Urological Private Department at Villa Maria Pia Hospital, Turin, Italy; Professor G. Muto, Professor of Urology and Head of Urological Department and Graduate Urological School at Campus Medical University, Rome, Italy; Professor F. Porpiglia, Professor of Urology and Head of Urologic Department and Graduate Urological School at Turin University, S. Luigi d'Orbassano, Italy; and Professor A. Volpe, Head of Urologic Department and Graduate Urological School at East Piedmont University, Novara, Italy.

A special thanks goes to A. Dezan who provided the anatomic drawings.

The author is particularly grateful to Alessandra Born of Springer for the continuous and valuable assistance with the editorial tasks.

Contents

Introduction

Some organs, such as the lungs, the kidneys, and the liver, are made up of lobes, which in the lungs and liver are clearly visible, but much less evident in the kidneys. The lungs and liver appear to have a lobated structure from the outside and shelter the internal functioning parenchymal segments. This function is inherent to all organ systems and can work independently due to the fact that it remains operative even when other parts of the lobe or the organ have been removed or are nonfunctioning as a result of illness. The segments have their own vessels, nerves, and aeration and secretion ducts, and as a result it is possible, when necessary, to remove the segment without causing any damage to the rest of the lobe (lung, liver). This leaves the organ sound and only deprived of the removed area.

In childhood, the kidney has an external lobated appearance, whereas in adulthood it is commonly compact or conglobate. In any case, the interior of its structure is composed of lobes, each made up of a minor calyx that receives the apex papillae of the pyramid surrounded by its own cortical envelop, which together form the renal segment. It is also possible to perform a lobectomy on the kidney, which is known as a renal segment ablation.

Some pathologies and diseases are temporary in that they represent just a stage in the process of an illness, others are definitive, referring to malformations or an irreversible pathologic situation with district localization, and are segmentary. In these cases, if surgical therapy is deemed to be necessary, segmentectomies or segmental resections are possible. In the kidney they are also called lobectomies or calicectomies.

These situations are perhaps rare but it is important to remember that rare does not mean nonexistent!

When and why those diseases or pathologies can be considered segmentary and thus necessitate renal segmentectomy and intrarenal plastic surgery is the topic of this book.

Readers will notice that the bibliography following some chapters occasionally appears old, as in the case of, for example, phylogenesis and the anatomic surgery of intrarenal operations and typical lobectomy techniques. For the section on phylogenesis I decided to report the source from which all the successive literature came, judging it inappropriate to ignore it. For the intrarenal surgery and lobectomy procedures I described in 1997, there are no significant notes or findings other than those published at that time by the Intrarenal Surgery Society, which are frequently cited in the book.

To better understand the topic, the book is divided into:

Part I: Pathologies and Diseases Representing Indications for Segmentectomy

Part II: Surgical Management

Part I
Pathologies and Diseases Representing Indications for Segmentectomy

Chapter 1
General Remarks

This part of Urology covers two inter-linked issues: Firstly, the study of pathologies and diseases that are located or potentially located in a single part of the organ, thus leaving the rest of it healthy and disease free; secondly, the study of surgical peculiarities in the targeted removal of part of the organ leaving the rest intact and functioning, known as segmentectomy. The value of the relationship between these two groups of study is clear if one wants to consider the pathological, clinical, and therapeutic aspects of each field.

This pathology will explain why pathologic phenomena or processes occur, and in some cases only temporarily, and remain in the specific part of the organ in which they started.

Clinical results will demonstrate if and when it is necessary to treat the disease or pathological processes in order to alleviate the issues or prevent them from getting worse. Therapeutic indications, in our case surgical, are part of the clinical discipline.

The surgical, segmentary treatment of the kidney consists of removing one or more renal lobes according to the manifestation and extent of the disease. Since the surgical technique begins by identifying the calyx in which the pathologic lobe opens, the lobectomy technique used is also called a calicectomy.

It is well known that it is possible to remove the affected part of the kidney through surgical procedures other than those specified above. This occurs in the case of small or

© Springer International Publishing AG 2018
S. Rocca Rossetti, *Managing Segmental Renal Diseases*,
DOI 10.1007/978-3-319-49721-1_1

medium-size tumors that are circumscribed and have no infil-
tration of the surrounding parenchyma. In this instance we
are speaking of partial renal resection.

It is thus timely to establish the difference between the
two kinds of procedures, both considered to be "nephron
sparing." The difference lies in both the surgical technique
and in the obtainable results. The surgical anatomy of segmentectomy is based on calyces, from which the name "calycectomy" is derived (Figs. 1.1 and 1.2). The calyx heads the

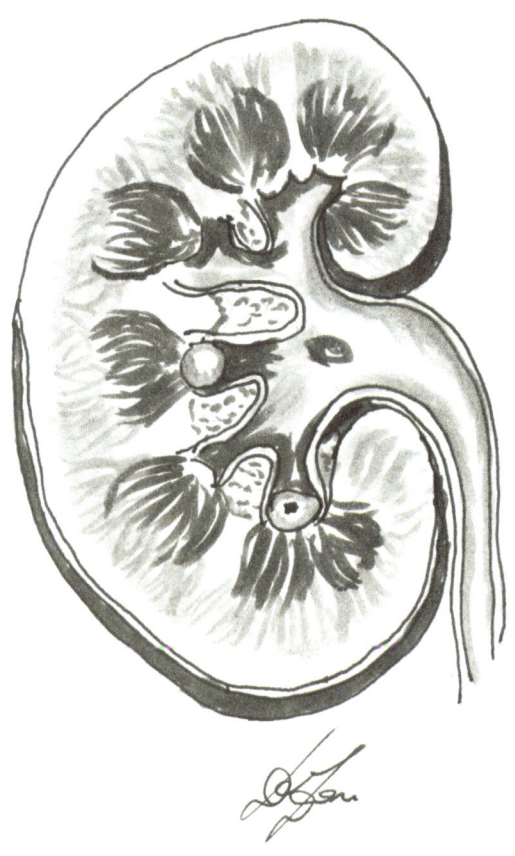

FIGURE 1.1 Renal lobation

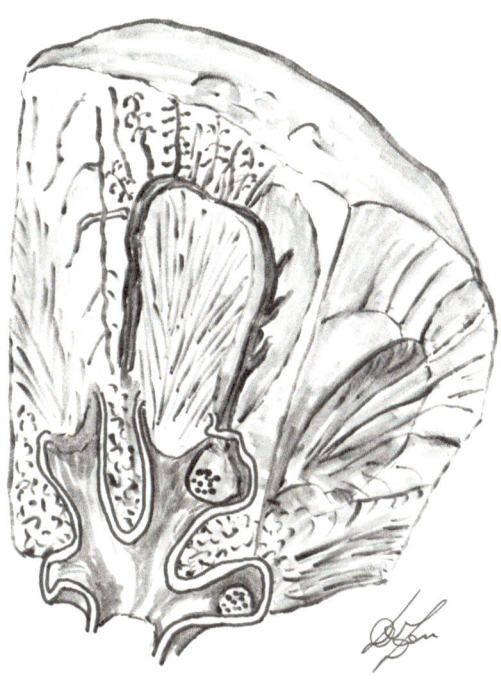

FIGURE 1.2 Renal lobes

segment or lobe that is to be removed; in order to reach the calyx one needs to enter the renal sinus and, using the major calyx as a guide, find the desired minor calyx. The calyx amputation and the traction on it favors the segmental paren-chymal delimitation that unloads in it and the consequent ablation.

While segmentectomy starts with intrarenal access (Figs. 1.3 and 1.4), partial nephrectomy starts from outside of the kidney, where the parenchymal incision is made just around the lesion that is to be removed, independent of whether the lesion is cortical, medullary, or calyceal (Figs. 1.5 and 1.6).

As far as results are concerned, segmentectomy leaves the rest of the kidney sound, missing only the removed lobe or

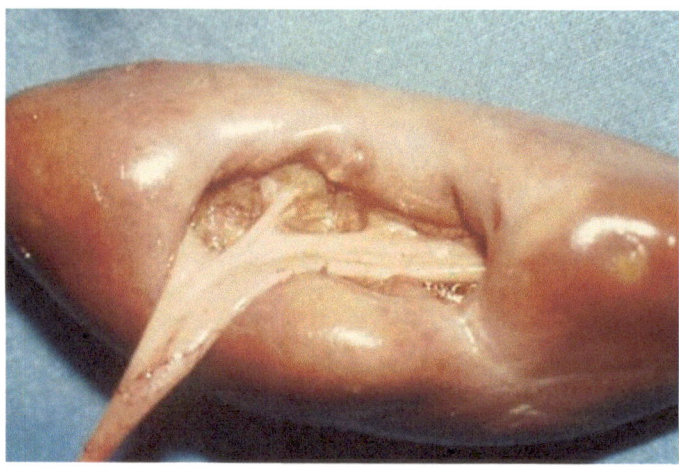

FIGURE 1.3 Renal sinus and calyces

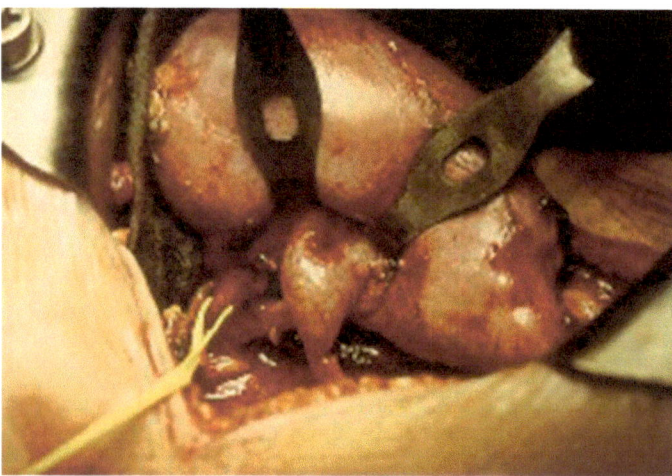

FIGURE 1.4 Preparation of the pelvis and calyces inside the renal sinus. Intraoperative photograph

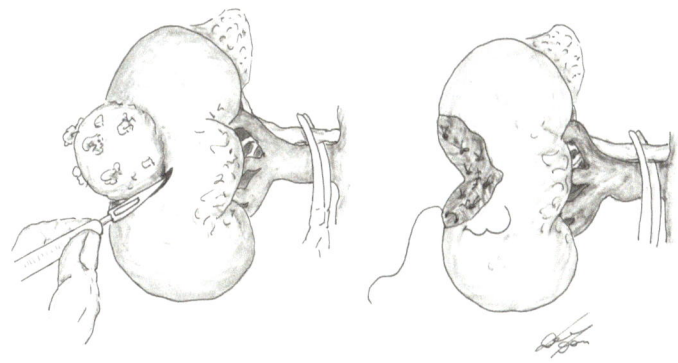

FIGURE 1.5 Partial nephrectomy from outside

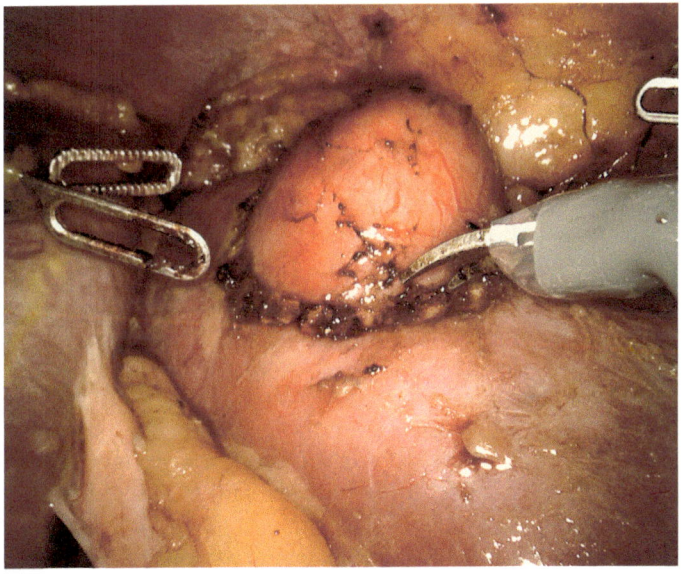

FIGURE 1.6 Robotic partial nephrectomy or tumorectomy, intraoperative photograph: Courtesy of Prof. A. Volpe

lobes. The reconstruction of closing the operated parts is done by moving them closer together using a capsular or nephrocapsular suture of the parenchymal lips.

Partial resection leaves a much bigger fibrotic scarring zone as a result of the reconstruction made on the area of the ablation; it most notably leaves a zone of non-functioning parenchyma, as it is deprived of calyces and is left without discharge. Naturally the indications are different for each technique. Since a partial nephrectomy is mainly indicated by circumscribed tumors or solitary cysts, it is much more frequently carried out than segmentectomy.

Historically speaking, the technical aspect of segmentectomy, also known as zonectomy, was so named after the identification of the anatomic meaning of a segment or zone. These words originated from the anatomic and anatomosurgical fields when the importance of avoiding the removal of the whole organ for a localized lesion was considered necessary. The question that arose was: why remove the entire organ when the pathologic lesion is limited to a single and sometimes small part of it, and the rest of the organ is sound and normal? The intrinsic structure, development, vascularization, and innervations of some organs were studied and the possibility of a positive answer to that question was found, together with techniques capable of removing a portion of the organ without interfering with the normal functionality of what remained of it. The advantage for the organism in those circumstances was clear.

The same consideration can be made, in our field, not only for the organ but also for the apparatus with which completely anatomically and anatomo-functionally independent areas can exist (see the chapter entitled Segmental or Nephroureterectomies).

In the second half of the last century the specific nature of the divisional structure of the lung was well known, and consequentially conservative surgery was suggested, for example pulmonary segmentectomies or zonectomies. It was in fact demonstrated that the lung is not only divided by scissures in lobes but also contains segments or zones, lined by slender

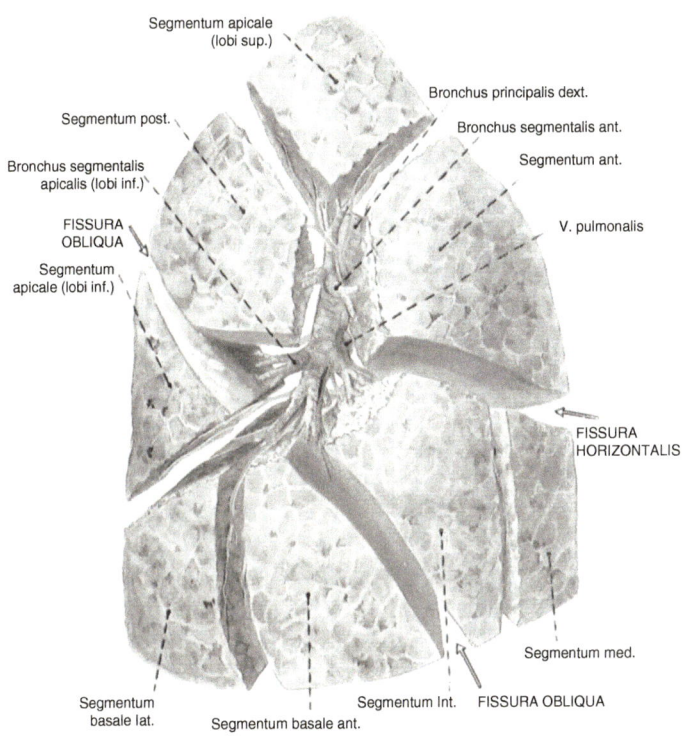

Segmentum apicale
(lobi sup.)

Bronchus principalis dext.

Segmentum post.

Bronchus segmentalis ant.

Bronchus segmentalis
apicalis (lobi inf.)

Segmentum ant.

FISSURA
OBLIQUA

V. pulmonalis

Segmentum
apicale (lobi inf.)

FISSURA
HORIZONTALIS

Segmentum med.

Segmentum
basale lat.

Segmentum Int.   FISSURA OBLIQUA

Segmentum basale ant.

FIGURE 1.7 Lung segments; from the Atlas of Anatomy, reprinted with permission of the Soc. Universo, Roma, 1971

connectival coverings. Each has an independent bronchial branch for air, and a proper nerve, artery, and vein, and can also function, if necessary, independently and autonomously from the rest of the lung (Fig. 1.7).

Embryonic ontogenesis has demonstrated that lung development is organized on the bronchus, that of the liver is organized on the portal venous branch, and that of the kidney on the calyx. As a result, segmental (pulmonary) resections, and then renal resections (also known as calicectomies), and eventually partial hepatic resections have been described.

It is thus evident that segmentectomy, or in our case calycectomy, is a surgical technique based on the anatomy that takes into account structure, clear boundary, vascularization, etc. As a consequence, after this kind of ablation the rest of the kidney or apparatus remains sound and is only deprived of the removed segment.

Alternatively, as has already been mentioned, a partial nephrectomy is also conservative surgery that saves the residual renal part that has been operated upon. It does, however, cause localized, ischemic scarring, and thus fibrotic damage with a decrease in kidney function, mainly because of bigger or smaller tissues being left without discharge. This reduction in functionality is certainly more considerable than that accompanying a segmentectomy.

In brief, renal segmentectomy is a surgical technique that is principally characterized by hilum access, sinus clear exploration, and lobar demarcation. It is not surgery that operates from outside of the kidney, but rather from the inside. It is thus unmistakably intrarenal surgery.

The organs that can withstand that kind of conservative surgery, based on the above-specified anatomic considerations, are those made on lobes, segments, or zones, such as the lungs, liver, and kidneys.

The human kidney, once completely developed, has a conglobate shape, like a single, compact mass. However, given its internal structure, it is really polylobate and polylobulated. The surgical technique in question here consists of localizing the lobe and removing it without harming the neighboring parts.

Considering the name, the word "calycectomy" stresses and underlines the concept of the organ's organization that is given to it by the calyx. The word "lobectomy" refers to the kidney being made up of lobes. Perhaps the word "lobectomy" is more appropriate for the current surgical terminology.

The lung segment represents the most typical segment shape. The bronchus, artery, vein, and nerve portion of the pulmonary parenchyma are bound by a very thin connecting envelope, known as the pleural scissure derivation.

Thus, returning to what has been said about the main principles of the topic we may say that: (a) The kidney segment (Fig. 1.2) is a renal lobe consisting of a calyx that collects the pyramid that is surrounded by a proper sheet of cortex. There is an invisible mesenchymal sheet dividing the cortical lobe from the neighboring one. (b) The renal vessels are called segmental, but since they are interlobar and not lobar, their segmentarity does not concern the surgical aspect of the segmentectomy. There are vascular areas of parenchyma that have nothing to do with segments; instead, they are important for partial nephrectomies. (c) Renal segmentectomy is a conservative intrarenal surgery that begins with larger renal sinus openings and that removes a single functional unit of the kidney, consisting of one or more lobes (Figs. 1.8 and 1.9), leaving the remaining parenchyma normally vascularized and drained by its collecting system (calyx or calyces). (d) A par-

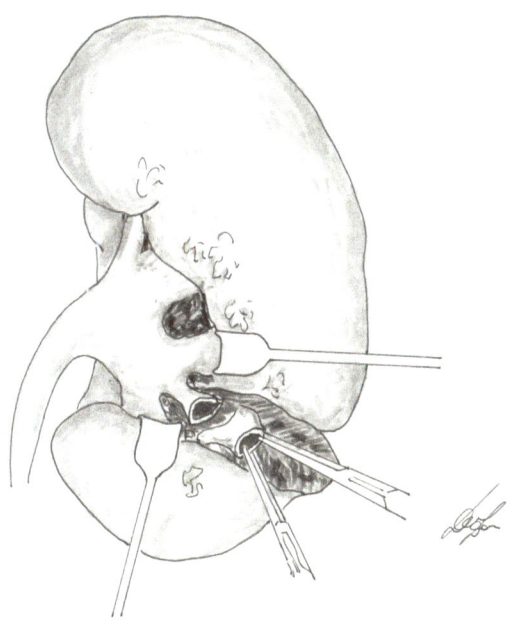

Figure 1.8 Lower pole lobectomy

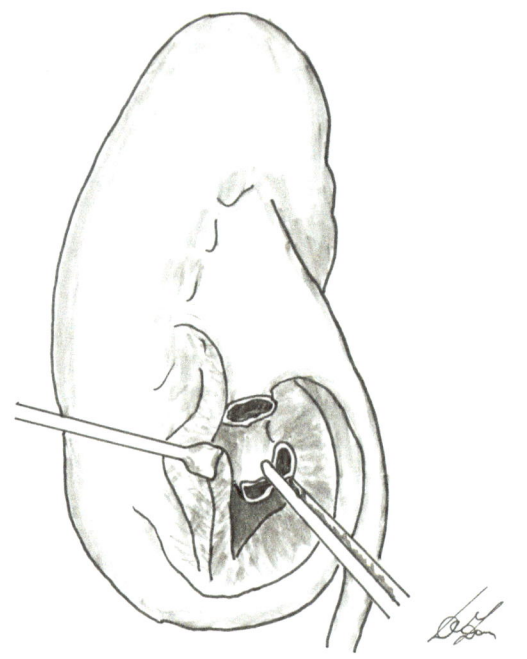

FIGURE 1.9 Lower pole lobectomy with open lower pole

tial nephrectomy, which is also a conservative surgery, removes a portion of kidney where the disease is located (i.e., tumor) independent of the vascularization and calyceal discharge. This means that the remaining parenchyma presents scars for devascularization, calyces without parenchyma, and parenchyma without calyces. (e) Renal segmentectomy, calicectomy, and lobectomy are synonymous; segmentectomy refers to the general concept of segment as specified above; calycectomy emphasises the influx of the calyx in the organization of the kidney; and lobectomy refers to the constitution of the internal lobe of the kidney.

The adult human kidney commonly appears compact and conglobate from the outside; early in childhood and sometimes also into adulthood it is the lobature that is so recognizable from the outside (Fig. 1.10).

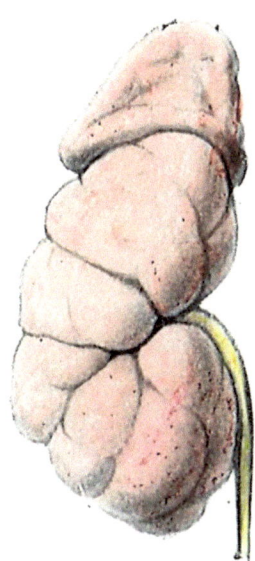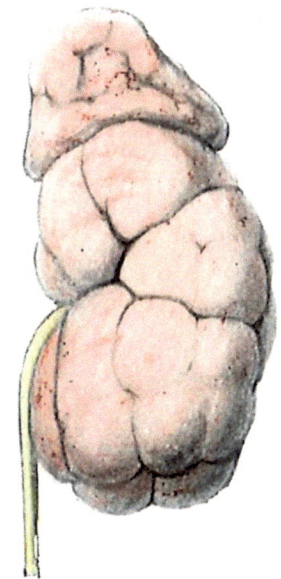

FIGURE I.IO Lobulated infant kidneys; from the Atlas of Anatomy. Reprinted with permission of the Soc. Ed, Universo, Roma, 1971

Finally, I believe it is appropriate to specify the particular meaning of the term "segment" reserved for what has been said here and will be said. In the medical literature, outside our surgical field, the term is used to signify "partial" or "part of it all" – as in the Latin segmentum from secare = sawing, cutting a part from a whole; thus we have: lumbar segmental instability; segmental colon pathology for constipation; segmental mastectomy; segmental Crohn's disease; segmental gene duplication; segmental nature of the choroidal vasculature; segmental vitiligo; segmental glomerolous sclerosis. A totally different meaning is given in this chapter and in those addressing the pulmonary and hepatic segmentectomy in which a segment is tantamount to an organ inside the organ with its own proper anatomic, functional, and surgical autonomy, removable without damaging the function of the whole organ.

Chapter 2
Kidney Stones

Much is known regarding the frequency, prevalence, geo-graphic manifestation, phylogenesis, etiology, physiopathol-ogy, clinical presentation, and therapy of kidney stones. Crystalline concretions are present in the kidneys of verte-brates and the equivalent excretory organs of invertebrates; the calcium constitution of the endoskeleton and exoskeleton creates the finite turnover and excretion of calcium, water conservation, and consequent low volume of urine. Thus, it is very difficult to keep calcium salts and other solutes in the urine solution since the laws of physiochemistry cannot be altered via biological evolution. Substances that promote and inhibit the calcium solution are well established in human urine, and their quality and quantity are of great importance, both in physiopathology and in a clinical setting. Urolithiasis is present in 0.5 % of US and EU populations, but its preva-lence has increased from 3.2 % to 5.2 % since the 1970s; blad-der stones have decreased notably in the last 20 years in developed countries. Stone recurrence remains at 50 % over 5–10 years and 75 % over 20 years; recurrence increases the probability of relapse and increases the amount of time between the two recurrences. These data are very important for what we shall go on to demonstrate here.

It is also known that it is not rare for stones to arise and grow in only one kidney, repeatedly, and for relapses to occur in the same area. It is certainly in a minority of cases in which this happens, but it does take place (no conclusive statistics on

© Springer International Publishing AG 2018   15
S. Rocca Rossetti, *Managing Segmental Renal Diseases*,
DOI 10.1007/978-3-319-49721-1_2

this could be found). The few authors that have addressed this topic have assumed nephrolithiasis to be the consequence of a previous illness in a part of the kidney (where it starts growing) that is capable of precipitating calcium salts, and thereby starts the stone-forming process [1, 2]. Renal stones can occur not only because of chemical processes or metabolic or genetic anomalies but also because of previous renal pathology. Recent research of various types has directly or indirectly supported the hypothesis on lithiasis occurring secondary to previous renal pathology. Firstly, so-called Darwinian medicine or evolutionistic medicine: According to the contentions of this recent branch of medicine the evolution of human phenomena occurs as a result of genes surviving so that those phenomena that have shown an advantage for the individual (food, reproduction) and the species are perpetuated. The usefulness of such (pleiotropic) genes is limited, depending on their purpose. Over time these adaptive features cease to be of any use to the organism and their presence can prove to be a source of harm. For example, it is supposed that calcium, a biophilic element that is indispensable for life, and a fundamental part of the skeletal and muscular system, is largely confined to bones, thanks to particular genes, so as to fortify them and provide them with the greatest possible resistance. This ensures that young individuals are given an advantage in enduring demanding functions like defense against predators, running, attacking, and so on. The genes that have survived are the strongest. The time scale for evolution is somewhat slower than for biology; so, in the case of calcium, the same genes once useful for surviving, over time (centuries, millennia) became risk factors for ectopic calcifications in arteries and other tissues. Calcium salt precipitation in the renal papillae and Henle's loop could therefore be the reason for lesions on which Randall's plaques grow.

An evolutionary anthropologist has ironically summarized the phenomenon with the phrase: "the price of not being eaten by the lion when you're young is paid by the risk of having heart attacks or arteriosclerosis when you're old" (or, in our case, renal stones) [1–5].

Clearly this evolutionary explanation for why stones grow and often relapse in only one kidney and area thereof can be objected to by pointing to the fact that nephrolithiasis is a disease most often found in young people, if not children. This leaves the pleiotropic genes in peace, which are probably involved in other more sophisticated situations.

Another consideration, pathogenetically linked to what has been said regarding prepapillary renal arteriole calcification, comes from research concerning extra-gastrointestinal lesions caused by *Helicobacter pylori*. *Helicobacter pylori* is presumed to be responsible for much urological pathology, such as chronic abacteric prostatitis, interstitial cystitis, and stone disease. Similar to what *Helicobacter* does to gastric mucosa – calcifications, arteriole thrombosis, and necrosis of mucosa epithelium, for example – it would create an analogous mechanism on the long Henle ansa and tubuli recti where the Randall's plaque begins [6]. Randall's plaques are invariably present in the former papillae of stones (and sometimes also in healthy people), and this structure is believed to be the nidus upon which calcium oxalate stones arise and grow. Microscopically the lesion seems to start in the basement membrane of the thin part of the loop of Henle, from where it expands through to the interstitium. Subsequently it involves renal tubules and vasa recta and eventually protrudes into the renal papilla epithelium. Biochemical studies have shown a transition from calcium phosphate to calcium oxalate in particular circumstances, such as the lesion in tubular lumen and in the collecting duct where Randall's plaques provide the platform for calcium oxalate crystals to form a heterogeneous nucleation and become a nephrolith. A correlation exists between plaques, urine volume, hypercalciuria, and the number of stones formed. The correlation is negative for urine volume and positive for hypercalciuria and the number of stones formed. The basement membrane calcifications are certainly early events. The true relationship between urine chemistry and the functional abnormalities that create the calcium phosphate deposition around the loop of Henle before the stone formation it is not clear.

Returning to the presence of peripapillary atrophy, arteriole calcifications in nephrolithiasis caused by *Helicobacter pylori,* Stoller et al. [13] appear to have confirmed the vascular etiology of the stone hypothesis. Randall's plaques could be the result of atherosclerosis, vascular injuries, or calcifications of the vasa recta.

Indeed, space medicine research on stone incidents in astronauts and on renal lesions in weightlessness also has valid contributions to make in understanding the way in which stones start on previous parenchymal lesions [8–10].

Today this topic attracts the attention of different extraction researchers, including those interested in intestinal microbiota variation. They are interested in investigating the reasons that stones often build in only one kidney and occasionally in only one specific part of that kidney. The research reported by Blaser and Falow [11] on the Bellini ducts and the long Henle ansa reaction to harm caused by arteriole calcification is particularly interesting in this regard. Epithelium cells should react with dedifferentiation in the presence of such anaplasia, acquiring the osteoblastic phenotype for metaplasia, followed by an increase in osteospecific protein osteopontin and a reduction in inhibitor crystallization factors like fetin A and Gla matrix. In doing so, matrix vesicula would create the crystal nucleation of calcium phosphate, which would transform later into calcium oxalate.

It is clear now that the problem of renal papillary arteriole calcifications is acquiring an important etiophatogenetic value in which the clinical relevance of stone recurrence in the same kidney deserves diligent investigation [7, 12].

When stones grow and relapse in the same kidney and in the same segment, the disease can be defined as segmentary.

In conclusion, among the various options currently available for the treatment of renal stones, segmentectomy is just one. It is, however, limited to non-frequent cases for which simple or complex stone removal would be insufficient to cure the patient since if part of the parenchyma is hopelessly damaged it would be a predictable source of relapses, if not worse, i.e., the formation of abscess.

Chapter 3
Renal Tuberculosis

Since 1967, renal tuberculosis has become less frequent and, as a result, surgery rare. In fact, compared to 15 years ago, there has been an increase in mild cases and conservative treatments. Renal and urogenital tuberculosis are always secondary or metastatic compared to pulmonary localization. The incidence of tuberculosis (TBC) among nations varies from 2 % to 20 % of the population, with an increase in proportion from industrialized to underdeveloped countries, where this infectious disease represents a real sanitary emergency. Comparative statistics from various institutions including the Health Ministry and National Institute of Statistics show a clear decrease in cases of TBC over the last 30 years, but they are not indicative of the situation regarding the urogenital localization of the disease, since non-infectious forms were not recognized for many decades after more general infectious TBC. Presumably the extra-pulmonary forms of TBC and, consequently the urogenital forms, have seen little increase in recent years. Among other things, renal TBC follows the first pulmonary or nodal infection by 15 or more years. This would explain at least partially the gap between the discovery of the two forms of infection.

It is worth revisiting the data of Gow [27, 28] from 1996, which show that of the total number of 3,000,000 global deaths from TBC, 3–4 % were from urogenital forms. Since menstrual blood examination has become routine, urogenital TBC in women seems to be much more frequent than in men [14].

© Springer International Publishing AG 2018
S. Rocca Rossetti, *Managing Segmental Renal Diseases*,
DOI 10.1007/978-3-319-49721-1_3

Among developed countries, Japan has the most new cases: 24.8/100,000 reported by the Japan Antituberculosis Association in 2003. During the same period Sweden had 5/100,000 and Kazakhstan 181/100,000, to show a snapshot of the geographical differences. As of 2004, genito-urinary TBC in Japan was not frequent, with a total of 144 cases, corresponding to just 0.5 % of the total forms of TBC [15].

At present immigration creates a great problem, considering how widely TBC is endemic and the areas from which immigrants predominantly come – they are a major source of infection and pharmacoresistence. The latter represents a serious problem, given the inadequate dosage and short period of treatment that is the result of the high cost of medicines. That can mean contagion from resistant bacteria and diseases that are difficult to treat. In Europe in 2014, 58,008 cases of TBC were reported (12/100,000) from 29 EU members and members of the European Economic Area, of which 76.2 % were newly diagnosed and 26.8 % were from unknowns; the latter percentage had increased from 19 % in 2005 to 27 % in 2014.

The World Health Organization in1999 reported that 17 million people were infected worldwide, 20 % of whom developed the disease, and with 8 million new cases per year (13–33 % in Western countries). Of the 8 million new cases, 2.8 million resulted in death, 40,000 of which occurred in developed countries and 2.7 million in underdeveloped (or developing) countries.

In 2006, 9.2 million new cases were reported worldwide, with 700,000 occurring in HIV patients. Of these cases, 1.5 million resulted in death, which equated to around 4,400 per day. The overall global incidence of TBC is still increasing, due to the 1 % increase in Africa.

These data suggest that without control TBC will kill 35 million people in the next 30 years and a total of 2 billion people will be infected, practically one-third of the world's current population. One in ten infected people will develop the disease and each infected patient will infect another 10–15 people each year. Multi-resistant TBC is present in 109 countries; in Eastern Europe 50 % of infected cases are multi-resistant.

In 2014 the Annual OSM Global Tuberculosis Report 2016 was published with a "Stop Tuberculosis Strategy" and an "End Tuberculosis Strategy" for reducing the 2015 mortality of infected person of 30 % to 15 % by the year 2030.

Fortunately Italy is a low-prevalence country with <10/100,000 inhabitants being infected. In 2006, 4,387 cases were reported, corresponding to 7.47/100,000 inhabitants, with a ratio of 1.47 male/female. Genito-urinary localization was 4.6 %.

The Report "Tuberculosis in Italy" of 3 November 2016, from the year 2008, shows that between 1955 and 2008 there was a reduction in the cases of TBC from 12,247 to 4,418. The crude rate went from 25.26/100,000 in 1955 to 7.4/100,000 in 2006. In the decade from 2004–2014 there were 4,300 cases each year, and 52 % of those were in non-Italian people (44 % in 2005, 66 % in 2014).

With regard to immigration, it is interesting to note that in big cities, like Milan, where there is a noticeable number of immigrants, the nationwide Italian ratio of 7/100,000 cases jumps to 20/100,000. Apart from the sheer number of cases, the immigrants create other problems, by way of pathology and care. In Germany, where there is perhaps the biggest immigrant community in Europe, Singh et al. have reported that among immigrants TBC was localized in the lymph nodes in 37 % of cases, in the bones in 20.5 %, in the central nervous system in 14.3 %, in the urogenital system in 8.5 %, in the lungs in 8.6 %, in the mediastinum in 5.7 %, and in the abdomen in 5.7 %. In 62.9 % of cases the chest X-ray was negative. It was clear that the common difficulties faced in recognizing the disease were intensified, not thanks to the unusual localization of it, but also because of its etiology and presentation. For example, the skin test was strongly positive until ulceration, the tuberculous interferon gamm release assay (IT-IGRA) was 100 % positive, while the nucleic acid complex of mycobacterium tuberculosis (NAAT) was only 35 % positive. In 91 % of cases mycobacterium tuberculosis was identified and myco-

bacterium bovis in 5.7 %. All reported cases were HIV negative. The delay in diagnosis was from 4–299 weeks. Suspected,
presenting, and prevailing symptoms were: lymphadenitis in
37.1 %, weight loss in 28.6 %, night sweats in 25.7 %, neuro-
logic symptoms in 22.9 %, cough and respiratory disorders in
14.8 %, bad back in 8.6 %, fever in 15.7 %, and other in 25.7
%. Urogenital localizations represented 3.18 % of cases.

All this considered, the modern danger posed by immigrants
with regard to TBC is high, both because of the frequency of
cases and the diagnostic delay. During the unfortunately long
period required to receive a positive diagnosis, every suspected
patient could go on to infect many people.

This summary data leads us to reflect on the evidence that
TBC in everyday medical practice is still a disease that is to
be considered as part of a differential diagnosis, particularly
in persistent (supposed) abacteric cystitis in persons who
have had contact with people originating from countries
where TBC is endemic. Of course it is worth remembering
too that "while the kidney is silent the bladder sings," old and
honest semeiotics.

So, why segmentary? The answer is in the renal TBC
pathology as the renal localization is hematogeneous. As a
consequence is cortical, diffuse, and nearly always bilateral.
In the vast majority of cases everything disappears very
quickly without leaving traces except for small, rare calcifications that are of no pathological significance. This step is
asymptomatic and devoid of bacilluria, since the glomerulus
is capable of filtrating water and crystalloids but not bacteria.
The glomerulus blood flow is too fast to allow bacilli stop and
grow, whilst the peritubular blood flow is not as quick. The
tubular epithelium is permeable enough and bacilli may
enter the interstitium and harbor there. The interstitial inva-
sion and harboring of TBC bacilli results in the formation of
TBC granuloma and its diffusion through the peritubular
vessels towards the papillary apex, where the ulceration of
the thin papillo-calyceal epithelium produces bacilluria. This
is the open phase of renal TBC. Diffusion in the excretory
system, the bladder, and eventually to the other kidney is
possible.

This pathologic succession could either occur simultaneously in different parts of the kidney or be limited to only one part where the papillo-calyceal ulceration enlarges, partially invading the pyramid with formation of fungo-caseous cavern. If the disease is left untreated over a period of time it will destroy a large part of the kidney.

The phase of the open renal TBC form in which the pelvis and ureter are still sound and in which only one or two papillae are invaded is the phase when the disease could be considered segmentary.

Renal segmentary TBC was excellently described by Semb [21–25], comparing the bronchopulmonary form to the renal one.

In segmentary localization, the removal of one or two pathologic lobes heals the patient, leaving the remainder of the kidney normal.

Patient complaints, the risk of cavern evolution, progressive enlarging of calcifications, and the lack of patency of the small calyces because of coartation or stenosis, form the basis for indication for segmentectomy. It is sometimes the case in these situations that when the calyx stenosis is total, the renal TBC can become a close form with an absence of bacilluria, and is consequently not easily recognized. Diagnosis can be difficult, but the absence of bacilluria does not preclude the possibility of a segmentectomy, since even close forms of TBC may be segmental. The same is true for the more rare renal tuberculoma [38–40].

We await the expected results of the OMS project: Eradicate Tuberculosis by 2050. However, conservative surgery is still indicated in segmental localization.

Chapter 4
Cystic and Mainly Malformative Diseases of the Kidney

Etiologic and pathogenetic data are useful if not necessary if we are to understand the segmentary nature of some malformative conditions, including cystic diseases of the kidney. As mentioned earlier, the development of the kidney and urinary tracts occurs over a series of stages that take place within a limited space and time. If this development is abnormal it can cause malformative nephrouropathies. The most serious of the malformative nephrouropathies is renal dysplasia: primitive tubules, embraced by stroma and a muscular collar surrounded by areas of nephrogenic mesenchyme together with undeveloped or less developed renal tissue and with non-renal structures like cartilage, muscles, and other structures, termed mesenchymal metaplasia [41, 42].

The human nephroureterogenetic process starts at about the fifth intrauterine week as a result of the connection of the ureteral bud of the Wolff duct to the metanephric mesenchyme. This develops into a definitive kidney. This mesenchyme triggers a process of gene transcription that induces on the one hand the prolongation of the excretory system, ureter, pelvis, and collecting ducts, and on the other hand the differentiation and proliferation of metanephric blastema cells. From that differentiation and proliferation some vesicles will form, that with prolongation, differentiation, and segmentation will make the nephron from the glomerulus to the distal tube.

© Springer International Publishing AG 2018   25
S. Rocca Rossetti, *Managing Segmental Renal Diseases*,
DOI 10.1007/978-3-319-49721-1_4

With regard to development time, it has been established that while the ureteric branching progressively decreases from week 15 onwards, formation of the new nephrons continues up to the 34th week and beyond.

Any alterations to these series of events, which are so intimately connected to one another, causes different anomalies depending on a number of issues. These issues include when the anomalies begin, the metanephric mesenchyme maturity, the tubular immaturity at the time, the different kinds of cyst formations and localizations, and the existence or absence of other excretory system anomalies. In terms of a timescale it would seem clear that, for example, the absence of the ureteric bud induction on the metanephrons causes agenesia, while stopping the ureteric branching and the epithelial differentiation would cause different kinds of dysplasia, ranging from a multicystic kidney to cortical or peripheral cysts [43].

Generally speaking, developmental failures are caused either by insufficient protoplasmic evolutive potential or, contrarily, by insufficient protoplasmic involutive potential. The consequence of the first cause is the developmental failure of the parenchyma and/or of the excretory system, such as agenesis, hypoplasia, and aplasia. A consequence of the second cause would be the excessive development and persistence of transitory elements that would ordinarily be destined to disappear. An absence of reduction in epithelial cell abundance in (solid) cords destined to become patent tubes, like the distal nephronic tubes, leaves them occluded, causing dilations or cysts (some readers may recall the Kemperer and McKenna theory on the involution failure of overabundance of primitive urinary tubules caused by the overabundance of nephrogenic blastemas, with respect to the numeric availability of collectors coming from ureterogenic gem; resulting in a lack of tubulo-collectorial meeting and consequentially cysts) [44].

Renal cysts are sac-like, epithelium-lined protrusions that have developed into renal parenchyma. They consist of liquid and start as expansions of pre-existing nephrons or collecting ducts of both embryonal structural elements. At this point they are a nephro-ureteric fusion anomaly. The inside liquid seems to derive from proximal and distal segments of primary nephrons. The epithelium that lines their surface is similar to that observed in the same segments of the nephron: functionally it retains the secretory activity. In some cases, over time, the cysts may lose all their connections with the original structures. Their pathogenesis is summarized in two predominant phenomena: epithelial hyperplasia of tubules and new or different secretive processes. Both contribute to the creation of endotubular hyperpression and the accumulation of similurinary liquid that develops tubular obstructions and cysts.

The aforementioned pathogenesis does not refer to the major numbers of renal cysts that occur in patients over a long period of time (5 and more years) that are treated with hemodialysis. In such circumstances cysts are generally small, subcapsular or at the cortico-medullary junction and, as part of the amyloid nephropathy, their content is liquid. In the majority of patients, the source of cystic liquid is not well understood. The obstruction of tubules seems to be caused by peritubular fibrosis or by calcium oxalate tubular occlusion. Given that the kidneys of dialytic patients are commonly small and retracted, their sudden enlargement indicates cystic complications, such as hemorrhage or tumors. Renal tumors, solid or papillary, frequently arise from the cystic epithelium and have a clear renal cell appearance [48].

In adults simple cysts are commonly acquired as a result of two principal factors: The first is the congenital presence of a small tubule diverticula, well illustrated by the microdissection technique [58], where the lesion starts. The second factor is precipitating substances and this is consistent with the obstruction of the urinary tract together with the normal involution of the basement membrane, typical of aging. With regard to aging, it is important to remember that in people under 40 years of age, simple renal cysts are rare, while from that age on almost 24 % of people have renal cysts in increasing numbers and size with age [56, 57]; 30 % of those cyst seem to be 2 cm or less, and are extra- or intra-parenchymal on abdominal CT.

The indications for renal segmentectomy (or partial nephrectomy) are exceptional for cystic diseases that concern only one single area of the kidney.

For completeness, it should also be noted that the same definition of a cyst could seem inaccurate compared to the total or partial excretory endorenal system dilation and their genesis. It is believed that the majority of kidney cyst formations (sporadic, acquired, congenital) originate from nephrons or collecting ducts either normally or not normally formed. An exception is multicystic dysplasia formed before nephron development from the lack of ureteral gem induction on the metanephric cap.

Much importance has been recently given to "ciliopathy" etio-pathogenesis for the manner in which it is involved in congenital cysts [59–61].

The sections below discuss only cystic diseases that, independent of their genesis, may occur as area- circumscribed and are therefore suitable for conservative surgery.

4.1   Cysts: Solitary, Typical, Atypical, Complicated

Surgical therapy for these cysts is not frequently indicated, is nearly exclusively for atypical or hemorrhagic or suppurated forms of puncture treatment [57]. In such cases segmentectomy, rather than extracapsular removal, can be considered when and if nearly all of the segment is involved (which is exceptional).

4.2   Multilocular Cyst or Cystic Nephroma

This is a rare kind of non-hereditary, organogenetic, dysembryogenetic, malformative disease, considered similar to benign neoplasia. It is relatively rare, but not excessively so given that recently five cases have been reported in Piedmont alone (an Italian region of 4,400,000 inhabitants) [62, 65].

Part of the renal parenchyma is replaced by a cluster of cysts that do not communicate between themselves and are not connected with the pelvis and calyces. A capsule envelops the cluster. It is always monolateral, and almost exclusively in women. What remains of the renal parenchyma is normal. There are often other malformations.

An infantile form also exists. It is generally considered to be one of the following: benign cystic Wilms' tumor, cystic nephroblastoma, or differentiated nephroblastoma. The diagnosis of this is generally on the basis of the presence of an abdominal mass.

Surgical treatment is by no means the rule, as especially in adulthood, patients are often symptomless, so surgery is reserved for large, complicated masses protruding in the abdomen. When the cyst bunch concerns one or more lobes, complicated by inflammation or hemorrhage, segmentectomy is indicated and the remainder of the kidney is considered normal and sound. Obviously preoperative or intraoperative tumor lesions have to be excluded.

As mentioned earlier, the cystic nephroma is often associated with other genitourinary malformations or the pathologies of different organs.

A possible, though very rare, association with endometriosis makes the diagnosis even more difficult, as in the case of C. Boccafoschi, in which this disease was associated with cystic lymphangioma involving the bladder and sigmacolon. The lymphangioma was presumably caused by a diffuse lymphatic obstruction at the pelvis level, which consequentially created lymphatic dilations and cysts. A type of lymphangioma was then at least partially acquired [65].

As mentioned above, since multilocular renal cysts may be considered neoplastic lesions, this was suggested as a more appropriate name [47]. This definition must be reserved particularly for cystic tumors that have been formed from entirely differentiated tissues, without blastema, or other embryonal elements. The designation of "nephroblastoma partially differentiated" defines cystic lesions as lacking in a solid, nodular area, while blastema or other embryonal tissues are present in cystic septa. They are not especially aggressive and never result in metastasis.

The reason for the lesion being known by such a variety of names, such as multilocular renal cysts, partially polycystic kidney, renal cystadenoma, polycystic nephroblastoma, differentiated nephroblastoma, and cystic nephroma, is the result of different etio-pathogenetic interpretations. Essentially there are two contrasting theories: neoplastic and dysplastic. The first seems to be more accredited today, supported by the fact that in dysplasic skeletal muscle, spots of metanephric undifferentiated blastema and immature mesenchyme such as that of nephroblastoma have never been found. The absence of typical elements of dysplasia, such as cartilage and embryonal ducts, support the neoplastic hypothesis.

The dysplastic-malformative theory relies on the idea of an autonomous vascularization that is independent from the renal vessels and originates in the lumbar vessels. This contention has appeared in the same literature and it assumed that cystic nephroma is a species of renal sequestration similar to pulmonary sequestration [70]. The latter is also a cystic malformation of the lung that does not communicate with the bronchial system and pulmonary vessels, but is nurtured by a systemic few vessels that it captures from the rest of the lung.

Another group of renal neoplastic cysts is the group of multilocular cystic renal-cell carcinomas, which represents a sub-group of renal cell carcinomas with proper macro- and microscopic characteristics. The features of these cysts include a variable quantity of neoplastic clear cells, with nuclear grade 1, and small or no mitotic activity. The cystic wall is fibrotic and often has no epithelium. Tumors are diploic at flux-cytometry and experience very low proliferative activity. Joshi et al. [47] believe this group of cyst to be a variant of low-grade clear cell renal tumors.

Finally, in order to avoid confusion, it is necessary to remember that the diagnosis of cystic nephroma is mainly based on the following characteristics: unilateral, isolated, multilocular, and unconnected to the pelvis or calices. The different cysts do not communicate with each other, and all the have a lined, defined epithelium, whilst normal and mature renal tissue is absent in them, and, importantly, the adjacent kidney is normal [69]. With regard to conservative therapy and then renal segmentectomy, it is very important to reach the diagnosis preoperatively, demonstrating that a good amount of normal paremchyma can be saved. One should also be aware of the possible presence of adenocarcinama or nephroblastoma foci in the lesion; however, this does not exclude conservative surgery with favorable results [67, 68].

4.3 Unilateral Segmentary Cystic Disease of the Kidney

About 50 cases of this disease have been published. They are differentiated from polycystic autosomic diseases (recessive or dominant) by the absence of familiarity, unilaterality, and segmentarity. This is a benign form that does not have the tendency to evolve into renal insufficiency and for which surgical treatment is not generally necessary, except in cases of space-occupying masses and pain [72].

The literature provides examples of nephrectomies being carried out due to the suspicion of the presence of a tumor, despite a good biopsy result. The anatomic specimen showed that the normal parenchyma was lesion free. Thus we now know that when a surgical indication exists, segmentectomy or another partial resection can be considered.

4.4 Cysts Associated with Renal Neoplasms

Two typical cyst-tumor associations are those of von Hippel-Lindau and tuberous sclerosis. Von Hippel-Lindau disease is transmitted by an autosomal dominant character. Cerebellar and retinal hemangioblastomas, pancreatic cysts and carcinomas, and renal cysts and tumors represent such a serious problem]. that the issue of the cyst itself is completely non-existent. Surgical treatment, which takes into account the complete or partial nature of the tumor, will be indicated. It is well known that maximum effort should be extended toward preserving the not-yet invaded parenchyma. For tumors that are less than 3 cm in size, nonsurgical renal-spearing strategies (radiofrequency, percutaneous ablation, and selective trans-catheter arterial embolization) have shown promise in short-term trials. For tumors that are more than 3 cm in size, conservative surgery, such as partial nephrectomy or even segmentectomy, should be considered.

In multiple tuberous sclerosis, which is transmitted via an autosomal dominant character, the hamartomas of the skin, brain, retina, skeleton, lungs, and kidneys are often associated with cysts. Sometimes the cysts are big and cause arterial hypertension. Indication for surgery is exceptional and nearly always based on the angiomyolipomas situation (present in 50 % of cases) and its clinical scenario is as follows: hematuria, hemorrhage, flank-loin pain, and life-threatening retro-peritoneal hemorrhage. Bleeding complications create an emergency and require urgent surgery. For this reason, con-servative treatment, which would otherwise always be desir-able, becomes in practice impossible. In that sense renal segmentectomy in cases of tuberous sclerosis represents just a theoretical indication.

It must be remembered that the first manifestation of tuberous sclerosis, though extremely rare, being unilateral, could be segmental cysts found in children, as in the case of the segmental cysts reported in 1997 by Wel Lara et al. [73].

Indeed, with regard to the relationship between renal cysts and tumors, interesting research is beginning to clarify the co-responsibility of proliferative activity of the cystic epithe-lium and genes regarding the induction of tuberous sclerosis. In this regard it was strongly suspected that the two major genes of tuberous sclerosis and polycystic kidney disease, TSC2 and PKD1, respectively, are adjacent in chromosome 16p, 13.3. It is on this basis that Sampson et al. believe that PKD1 has a role in the etiology of tuberous sclerosis [79].

Apart from von Hippel Lindau and tuberous sclerosis diseases, with regard to the cyst/tumor association, clinically the problem of identifying the presence of neoplastic tissue in cysts appears predominantly in complex cysts, where the occurrence of malignancy is greater. Imaging with radiologic follow-up and guide biopsy is able to reach the correct diagnosis and avoid unnecessary surgery in 39 % of cases of cystic renal masses, the second category of Bosniak, according to Hansinghani et al. [80]. Apart from complex cysts, CT imaging shows some cysts with unusual content, now known as hyperattenuating renal masses. These cysts are wholly or predominantly filled with CT attenuation, higher than the surrounding parenchyma. Protein or iron concentration, hemorrhage, colloids, infections, and occasional iodine accumulation are the most frequent reasons for the hyperattenuation of simple cyst content. Hyperattenuating renal masses may also be constituted by hematoma, vascular aneurysm, malformations, malignant cysts, benign hyperattenuating cysts, and other hyperattenuating solid masses. As a consequence, the importance of recognizing the etiology and pathogenesis of the lesion is essential for correct clinical diagnosis. In the majority of cases the cysts are benign, and it must be emphasized that when neoplastic, the small cysts, with homogeneous enhancement hyperattenuating, should be considered to be of benign origin [80, 81].

4.5   Multicystic Segmentary Dysplastic Disease

A few dozen cases reported in the literature of non-hereditary multicystic dysplastic infantile subunits were diagnosed by ecography, TAC, and MRI. Some of these were reported in young patients and consisted of multiloculated, multiple cysts of different sizes. They did not communicate, were commonly localized at the polar level, did not hold the contrast, and did not intercept intercystic solid mass. The remainder of the kidney may be normal or experience inflammatory phenomena, generally due to vesico-uretero-renal reflux. The excretory system could be normal or duplicated.

This type of renal dysplasia has an incidence of 1/4,300 live births and seems to be due to an inhibition of ampullar activity in the ureteral bud and its inhibition in the mesonephric blastema. Consequently there is little contact between the ectopic uteteral diverticulum and the metanephros. An early *in utero* obstruction and a consequent urinary stasis with cyst formation has also been hypothesized. There is a frequent association with other abnormalities of the urinary system.

The differential diagnosis includes the multicystic segmental kidney, benign multilocular cyst, multilocular cystic nephroma, and cystic Wilms' tumor. The absence of unilaterality and familiarity are enough to exclude polycystic infantile and adult diseases. The lack of functioning solid masses and absence of contrast at the cystic level excludes cystic nephroma, multilocular cysts, and cystic Wilms'. The preoperative diagnosis is then mainly based on an exclusively nonfunctioning cystic mass with benign characters. The anatomic specimen shows non-communicating cysts of various sizes, the absence of neoplasia, conspicuous fibrosis, and chronic inflammation of the tubules, surrounded by primitive characteristic mesenchyme.

Being segmental, this disease could allow for a conservative treatment and therefore segmentectomy [88].

4.6   Medullary Cysts

There are two forms of medullary cysts: sponge medullary kidney and familiar nephronoptisis cysts. Only the former can be monolateral and occasionally arise in only one or two pyramids, i.e., segmentaries. The pathology concerns collecting, thick, obstructed ducts. The parenchyma is remarkably modified by multiple, generally small cysts containing stones and by rather intense fibrosis. There are frequent associations with other somatic anomalies, such as congenital emihyper-trophy, and Marfan and Ehlers-Danlos syndromes.

Although exceptional, a mass-like, localized medullary sponge cyst may appear as a tumor [100, 101].

Normally the disease remains asymptomatic and there is no need for any treatment besides a large intake of fluid in order to prevent stones.

When the disease is segmentary and only one or two pyra-mids are involved, surgery that could in fact prove to be complicated, but may be indicated. Segmentectomy could be the choice, since the lesion side is generally polar.

4.7   Cysts of Renal Sinus

These cysts are commonly treated by punction. In case of surgery intrarenal sinusal access is compulsory, but the seg-mentectomy has no indications unless it is otherwise required by the existence of parenchymal pathologies [103].

Chapter 5
Other Potential Segmental Pathologies

5.1 Renal Hyperplasia and Hypoplasia

These types of pathology do not need conservative surgery and segmentectomy. The only exception is Ask-Upmark kidney or segmental hypoplasia. This maldevelopment forms cortical scars, sinking, and wrinkling of the underlying pyramids, and dilation of relative calyces. Histologic examination of this abnormal metanephric differentiation shows microcysts and the absence or glomerular paucity. Urethral valves and vescicorenal reflux, with or without infection, frequently coexist. This demonstrates the acquired maturation of the lesions, although already present in intrauterine life. Obviously conservative surgery and segmentectomy could be considered when the segmentary form of the hypoplasia is associated with normal unaffected parenchyma. It is also obvious that prior to renal conservative surgery, any other malformations (urethral, ureteral) must be corrected, if present [104–109].

5.2 Special Infections and Inflammations

Some types of pyelonephritis could arise mainly or exclusively in a single area of the kidney. In these cases, when surgery is indicated, renal segmentectomy could be the best choice.

© Springer International Publishing AG 2018   37
S. Rocca Rossetti, *Managing Segmental Renal Diseases*,
DOI 10.1007/978-3-319-49721-1_5

Among those conditions, pyelonephritis, the xanthogranu-
lomatos type, also known as renal pseudotumor, has been
observed in thousands of cases worldwide despite not being
a frequent disease, and has attracted the attention of urolo-
gists for presentation, modality, and treatment choice, which
often proves to be surgical.

As is known, it is a granulomatous form with typical foamy
cells that can evolve silently, but that routinely manifests with
symptoms of infection, general weakness, toxicosis, and local
and general complications that can sometimes be very serious, such as septic syndrome, amyloidosis, parietal and vis-
ceral fistulae, renal vein thrombosis, and so on. Bilateral
forms are exceptional. The regional or segmental forms give
rise to a strong suspicion of the presence of a tumor, due to
the unaffected integrity of the parenchyma. Thus a careful
differential diagnosis, both clinical and radiologic, is necessary. The persistent or relapsing history of a urinary infection,
the bacterial peculiarity (proteus, pseudomonas, coli), the
typical urinary cells, the associated urinary stones, the
sequence of previous sonographic examinations, as well as
the precision of imaging tests are all useful or even indispensable for obtaining the correct preoperative diagnosis.

When surgical conservative treatment seems necessary,
segmentectomy could be considered given the good results
that can be obtained with regard to the healthy parenchyma.
This is the case in infantile forms or in medullary localized
forms in adulthood.

Though exceptional, some forms of conservative surgery
for renal xantogranulomatosis caused by bilharzia have been
described. Routinely renal lesions of bilharziosis consist of
ureterohydronephrosis due to vesico-ureteric parasitic inva-
sion. Nevertheless, cases of true parasitic renal xantogranulomatosis due to schistosomas are rarely missed. In a minority
of those reported cases a good portion of the kidney was
sound, thus allowing for conservative surgery [113, 114, 117].

5.3   Other Endorenal Pathologies: Hydrocalyx

This malformation consists of the dilation of a calyx with consequent tributary parenchyma destruction, caused by the compressive ischemia, which could also affect the neighboring parenchyma. The hydrocalyx is drained by the obstructed infundibulum. It is still a matter of disagreement whether or not the congenital forms are due to calyceal neck achalasia and if the acquired form could be caused by something capable of creating an obstruction such as prolonged spasms, fibrosis, etc. Hydrocalyx is clinically relevant only for complications, such as hemorrhage, infections, and painful stones.

According to the nature of the symptoms and the seriousness of the renal harm, when endoscopic treatment fails, partial ablation is indicated and typically segmentectomy as well.

5.4   Calyceal Diverticulum

This maldevelopment concerns a small calyx eventration lying within the renal parenchyma and communicating with the main collecting system through a narrow channel. The diverticulum is lined by a transitional epithelium, which appears to be because of the absence of reabsorption of third- or fourth-generation ureteric branching. It is often asymptomatic and clinically irrelevant, but it could be a sign of obstruction, stones, or suppurative flogosis requiring surgical treatment. Endoscopic, percutaneous, or minimally invasive pathways are frequently available, but if the corresponding renal lobe is hopelessly compromised, segmentectomy should be the treatment of choice.

5.5   Megapolicalycosis

This malformation is a medullary papilla hypoplasia with consequent dilation, expansion, and apparent multiplication of calyces without obstruction. The pelvis and ureters are normal. The condition is due to an anomaly in the development of the ureterogenic blastema in the collecting ducts. It would seem to be supported by late channeling of the high ureter, to which the ureteral gem branches are connected via the metanephric blastema. The delay creates some sort of obstruction of primitive glomeruli when they start to work. According to the general concept of the ureterogenic theory, the epithelial structure also induces the support of scaffolding organization. Consequently the failure of the uretrogenic blastema prevents development of the pyramidal structure.

Megapolicalycosis is thus congenital. The male/female ratio is 6:1, and the White population are most commonly affected. In males it is bilateral and in females it can only be segmentary.

The medullary portion is hypodeveloped with a crescent or sickle shape. The collecting ducts are not dilated but are shorter than normal and are transversely oriented compared to the cortico-medullary junction. The renal function remains normal.

In the majority of cases the disease is discovered casually. Surgical indication is quite rare or exceptional, as it is reserved for local, sectorial complications like infections or stones. Segmentectomy involves improving the outcomes of those lobar complications.

5.6   Infundibulo-Pelvic Dysgenesia (and Fraley Syndrome)

An infundibulo-pelvic stenosis is probably caused by an anomaly in the ureteral gem. It is often associated with a cystic dysplasia of the kidney. The stenosis grading is variable.

A focal form that involves only one or two calyces may exist, but commonly the disease is bilateral and associated with vesico-renal reflux.

Histologic examinations of infundibular renal stenosis [38, 43] have shown a hyperplasia of smooth muscles within the submucosa with scattered rare interstitial spindle cells that are CD117 positive, similar to the cells responsible for peristaltic pacemaker activity of the gastrointestinal tract. The presence of CD117 cells suggests that the calyceal narrowing is due to renal hyperplasia and not to leiomyomatosis. However, which of them is the hyperplasic stimulus is unknown.

This condidion is frequently asymptomatic and the diagnosis is achieved on the basis of the presence of hypertension, infection, and lumbar pain.

An indication for a conservative surgery, such as a segmentectomy, is put forward based on its localization, renal function, and symptoms.

Conversely, due to the superior calyx dilation being the longest, it is the only one to be caused by a vascular compression, which is more frequently arterial, and also known as Fraley syndrome [79], for which normally there is no question of a segmentectomy (Fig. 5.1).

5.7   Reno-Ureteric Segmentectomies

There are conditions of the reno-ureteric duplicate collecting systems in which the ablation of one of the two segments is necessary. The reason for surgery is commonly aplasia or another pathology of the parenchyma, which has been drained by the supernumerary excretory pathway share. Such malformative conditions are generally recognized in childhood and, if complicated, surgery (strictly that of ablation) is not compulsory.

The collecting system duplicity occurs in just under 1 % of births and in the majority of cases it is asymptomatic. It may be complete or partial in the pelvis and ureter, depending on

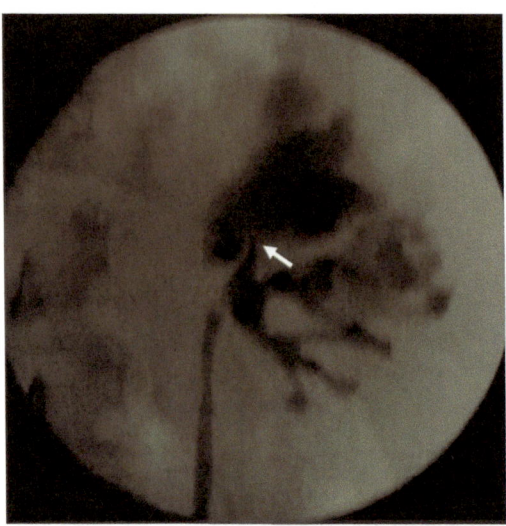

FIGURE 5.1 Abdominal CT scan suggesting the presence of a crossing vessel at the left upper pole infundibulum resulting in a hydronephrosis. Courtesy of Prof. F. Porpiglia

whether the ureteral gem branched to join the metanephric blastema at an early or late stage in development. It seems to be a dominant autosomal form with poor penetrance. In 12 % of cases it is associated with other urinary anomalies, 50 % of which are on the same side and to which the causal role of complications and related symptoms are attributed. In a majority of cases (88 %) there are no true complications.

In incomplete duplicity, the so-called yo-yo phenomenon [158–160] may cause back pain or infection. It can be that the systole of one ureteric branch is occurring simultaneously to the diastole of the other branch, which results in incomplete emptying and dilation of diastolic refluxing segment. In these circumstances the reflux is pathogenetically very important, especially the intrarenal one. Pyelolymphatic, pyelovenous, pyelotubular, and pyelointerstitial systems may have septic (the former two) or phlogistic and sclerotic (pyelotubular) complications. Intrarenal reflux, the seriousness of which is associated with local circulatory conditions [89], is especially frightening for malformed kidneys. (The reflux nephropathy is a severe complication of the urinary collecting system pathologies, which at first may not seem to be important. Experimental research demonstrates the conditions under which intrarenal reflux may become severe; among these intrarenal blood pressure and pyelic pressure deserve careful attention). Obviously in these cases a timely diagnosis allows for conservative treatment of pyelo-pyelo or uretero-uretero anastomosis.

The double district ablation or the ablation of a ureteric portion could be called a segmentectomy. The word segmentectomy could apply to the pre-ureteric vena cava (the so-called retrocaval ureter) or to regional, intrinsic, and ureteric pathologies, which necessitate exeresis. The word segmentectomy is lexically correct, but not in a urologic sense, since it could lead to ambiguity. For example, on the one hand such ablation leaves the remainder of the urinary system sound and functioning, but on the other it does not refer to a specific segment. In cases of double district ablation there are two organs, an aplastic or pathological kidney and a ureter, thus not one or two segments. In case of partial ureterectomy it is a matter of removing the part of the organ in which organogenetic individuality does not fall within the segmentariety concept.

For those reasons it must be assumed that double district and partial ureterectomies are not segmentectomies according to the above definition.

Part II
Surgical Management

Chapter 6
Organisation of Kidney and Urinary Apparatus

It is well known that renal development occurs in three stages, each one countersigned by a transient, tubular organ. These stages are pronephros, mesonephros, and metanephros. To avoid spending too long describing this topic, here we will only consider data specifically to do with the subject of segmentation.

In very low stages of the zoological scale there are tubes that are for the external discharge of toxic materials. In invertebrates, like some worms (annelid), there are nephridia in each disc or body segment, which are able to excrete the toxic portion of protein metabolism. At a higher level of the zoological scale, it becomes necessary to also eliminate excess water from the body. This new function is performed independently from the excretory function. The filtration ducts run independently and are isolated compared to the excretory ones. Only vertebrates have a true and proper organ for those two (and other) functions. The kidney does not discharge products outside the body, but inside at cloacal level (Fig. 6.1). The phylogenetic transition of the urinary apparatus is evident in sharks, in which the nephridia of every somite does not open outside but flows into a discharging duct (Wolff duct) that opens in the cloaca. The fusion of those two structures and functions in a single organ are seen clearly in reptiles, birds, and mammals.

The pronephros, or primordial kidney, works only in fish, with nephridia for every somite in the body. It is the first of

© Springer International Publishing AG 2018   47
S. Rocca Rossetti, *Managing Segmental Renal Diseases*,
DOI 10.1007/978-3-319-49721-1_6

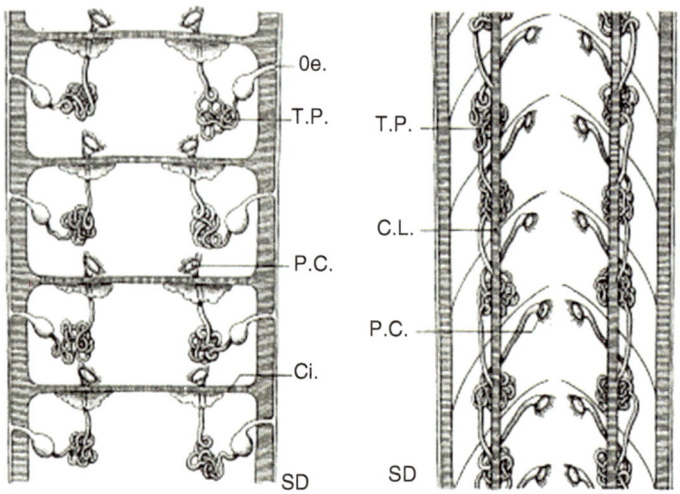

Oe.
T.P.   T.P.

C.L.

P.C.

P.C.

Ci.

SD   SD

Figure 6.1 Renal phylogenetics; nephridia of invertebrates: external discharge (*left*); vertebrate (shark) kidney (*right*); internal cloacal discharge and Wolff duct; reprinted with permission of O. Doin et al. Edit. Paris, 1914

three similar tubular organs involved in the genito-urinary apparatus. The pronephros disappears in all vertebrates and is substituted by the mesonephos. The mesonephos is definitive in some animals, such as amphibians, while it is intermediate in man and in other superior animals (mid kidney). It transforms in shape and function only partially and is replaced by the metanephros, which is the last of the three similar tubular organs to be transformed. The metanephros is located in the pelvic zone and will evolve into the definitive kidney.

In mammals the definitive kidney works to filtrate and excrete simultaneously. The two tubular structures are separated and dislocated over a very short period of time in the metanephric evolution and then in quick succession they come together after forming the definitive morphological and functional unit for filtration and excretion. This ensures that products are ejected from the body and a constant water balance with the normal amount of water in fluids and tissues is maintained.

In man the transformation of metanephros in the definitive kidney occures within the fifth week of intrauterine life (i.e., fetal life) and it is complete at the second month of gestation. This increase and improvement in the kidney lasts beyond birth.

The aforementioned transformation is countersigned by two fundamental stages that concern kidney segmentation. At the cloacal level a diverticulum appears from the Wolff duct (residue from the pronephros and mesonephros duct). This is initially solid and later channeled, growing postero-laterally until it reaches the metanephrogenic bonnet or metanephric blastema of the posterior mesodermic derivation. The meeting of those two structures induces a strong stimulus of differentiation with S-shaped tubular formations, which spread cranially embracing capillary branches, and primitive arterious glomeruli. Distally they increasingly grow in the direction of the Wolff duct diverticulum, which is now completely patent and tubular. The superior end of this tube, after having spread, enlarges in ampullary form and creates the primitive pelvis. It divides into primitive major calyces (Bellini collecting ducts), eventually becoming nephrogenic structures, which come from the metanephrogenic cup [166–168].

Phylogenetic studies show the formation of several renal lobules, each one containing parenchyma drained by a calyx, and vascularized by one or two arteries and veins (frog kidney). In other animals, such as young elephants, a lobar constitution is recognizable (Fig. 6.2).

In the majority of animals, man included, the kidney appears compact with the external area being generally smooth and conglobate. However, the intrinsic structure of mammal kidneys reveals the parenchyma is formed by an external part, the cortex, which encloses the internal part, the pyramid or medulla, and is drained by a minor calyx. The cortex contains glomeruli and tubules while the pyramid contains only tubules. The whole pyramid, together with the sur-

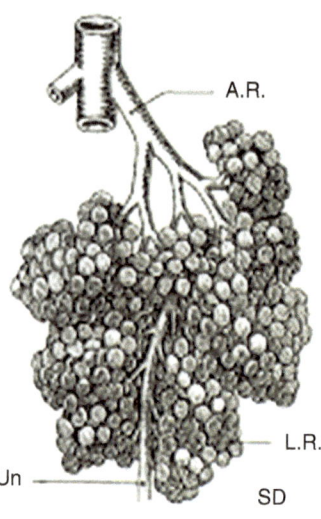

FIGURE 6.2 Lobulated kidney of dolphin; reported with the permission of O. Doin et al. Edit. Paris, 1914

rounding cortex, and the discharging calyx constitute a lobe that is not externally visible. A very thin connective layer with some smooth muscle cells invisibly separates one lobe from its neighbors [169–171]. Two, or in exceptional cases more, pyramids may be drained by the same calyx, especially at the poles. Commonly in human kidneys there are 12 or 13 lobes (Fig. 6.3).

Phylogenetic and anthropologic studies show that the renal medulla is only divided into many lobes in fish, aquatic mammals, and in those terrestrial mammals that were derived from an aquatic ancestor. In this regard, the M.F. Williams paper (2006) on "Morphological evidence of marine adaptation in human kidneys" underlies the evolutionistic aspect of this fact stating: "Amongst primates, kidneys normally exhibiting lobulated, multi-pyramidal medullas are a unique attribute of the human species" [164]. Although kidneys that are naturally multi-pyramidal in their medullary morphology are rare in terrestrial mammals, kidneys with lobulated medullas occur in elephants, bears, rhinoceroses, bison, cattle, pigs, and

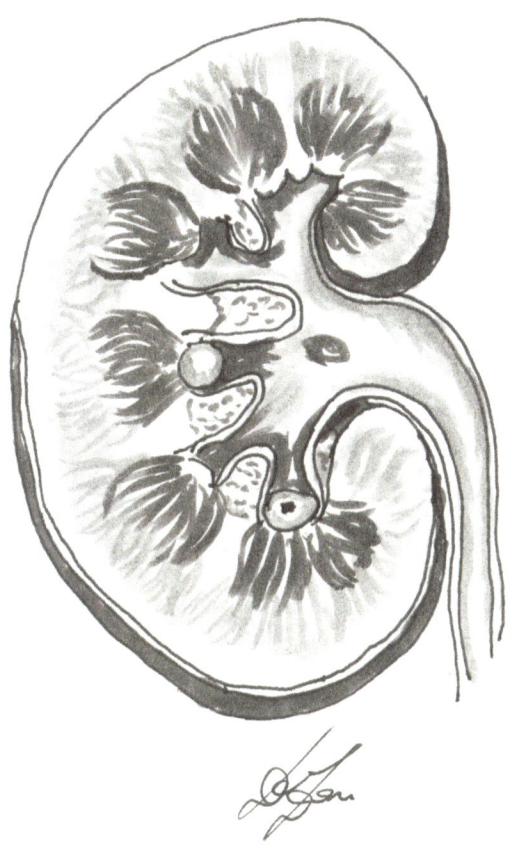

FIGURE 6.3 Renal lobation

okapi. However, kidneys characterized with multi-pyramidal medullas are common in aquatic mammals and are nearly universal in marine mammals. To avoid the deleterious effects of saline water dehydration, marine mammals have adaptively thickened the medullas of their kidneys, which enhances the ability to concentrate excretory salts in the urine. However, the lobulation of the kidney's medullary region in marine mammals appears to be an adaptation to expand the surface area between the medulla and the enveloping outer cortex in order to increase the volume of marine dietary-induced hypertonic plasma that can be immediately processed for the excretion of excess salts and nitrogenous waste. The substantial loss of genetic variation in humans relative to other hominoid primates, combined with the apparent isolation of early Piocene human ancestors from particular retroviruses that infected all other African primate species, may suggest that such a semiaquatic marine phase, during the emergence of Homo, may have occurred on an island off the coast of Africa during the early Piocene era.

This is an interesting evolutionistic aspect of the human renal lobulation [164, 165].

Returning to the main topic, kidney vascularization is in accordance with segmental renal organization in the sense that the vessels are distributed to specific groups of parenchymal areas in anterior faces, posterior faces, and polar zones, but not to the 11 or 13 lobes of the kidney. The vessels are known as "segmental," but this definition does not suit the concept of the proper segment specified above, which focuses on the surgical aspect of lobe excision. The renal arteries and veins are indeed interlobar, not lobar.

In this regard Fred Graves's precious research on renal vascularization [164] has confirmed a sectorial renal vascularization that does not relate to segments. The research is certainly useful as far as nephrostomies and common partial nephrectomies are concerned, but not for specific segmentectomies, like lobectomies or calicectomies.

Exploiting the fact that arteries and veins are distributed to certain well known areas, surgically cutting the parenchyma between two adjacent surfaces will find less vascularized tissue, even if it is not especially ischemic. The surgical method of anatrophic nephrostomies is based on this type of research [173]. Thus the F. Graves standardization of renal vessels is of great importance for kidney operations, but the renal vascular area is not a renal segment or lobe. In human beings the lobe lost the lobar vascularization found in frogs and dolphins. Because of its ascent from the pelvis to its current position, the renal lobe was organized according to calyceal induction, while the vessels appeared and disappeared according to the kidney's position at that time. We can thus conclude that the surgical technique of segmentectomy is based on the calyx and not on the artery or vein.

This is a topic that I have discussed many times with my great friend Fred Graves.

Chapter 7
Surgical Anatomy of Urinary Segments and Operative Surgical Aspects

In the urinary tract the true segments are identifiable in renal lobes, in supernumerary kidneys, and, in theory, in complete or incomplete reno-ureteric duplicity (multiplicity). Those structures correspond to the previously described segment concept: They have proper functional autonomy and proper vascularization and innervation, and their removal, correctly executed, leaves the rest of the apparatus unscathed.

Even if one segment is removed (lobectomy) the portion of the kidney that is saved (the parenchyma and calyco-pyelic excretory system), is left normal and healthy (Figs. 7.1, 7.2, and 7.3).

7.1 Renal Segments, Calycectomy, Segmentectomy, Lobectomy

As described earlier, the kidney is organized on a calyx that causes it to differentiate into secreting parenchyma once it reaches the metanephrogenic cup. Those tubules keep extending until they join the Bellini collecting ducts of calyceal derivation, of which they are a continuation. The minor calyx with its tributary pyramid and the surrounded cortex make up the renal lobe. From outside, with the exception of fetal lobature persistence (Fig. 7.8), lobes are not visible and hence not identifiable. However, penetrating the renal hilum and

FIGURE 7.1 Outline of lower pole lobectomy

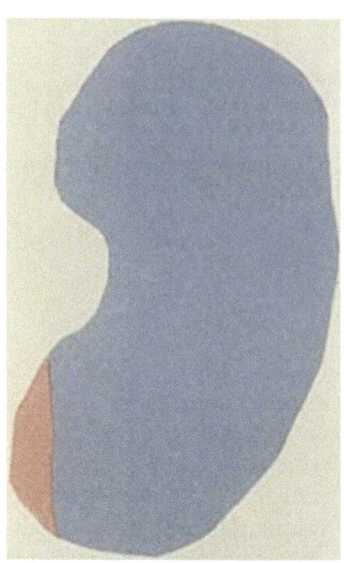

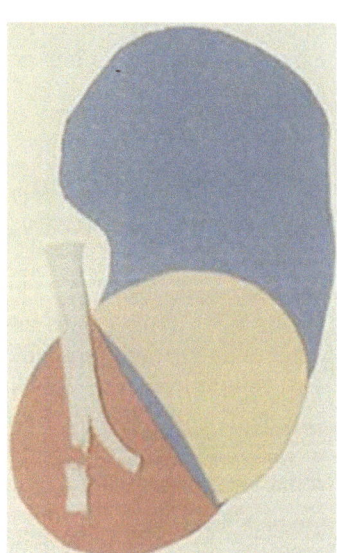

FIGURE 7.2 Outline of lower pole lobectomy: open lower pole

FIGURE 7.3 Outline of upper
pole bilobectomy, showing the
result

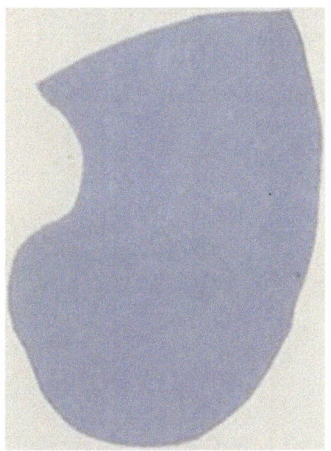

following the major and minor calyces it is easy to reach the
renal papilla or pyramid apex through the loose connective
tissue of the renal sinus. Having done this, through a small
targeted nephrotomy, it is not difficult to identify the lobe
and remove it correctly, by following each side of the pyramid
edges inside the cortical tissue that divides one pyramid from
the next (Figs. 7.4, 7.5, 7.6, and 7.7). Hemostasis occurs little
by little as meeting vessels branch from the interlobar vessels
and penetrate the pyramidal parenchyma and the vessels of
the small interposed cortical tissue near the capsule. When
and if the vessel's small mouths are identified, clamping with
a mosquito clamp is suitable and not difficult. This is followed
by ligature or suture. For local, pathologic situations a severe
hemorrhage could occur. It is better to clamp the renal artery
or its tributary branch for that part of the kidney earlier. The
clamping could be associated with renal cooling. In cases of
surgical complexity, large areas of inflammation, or sclerosis,
one could expect the ischemia to last more than 20 min.

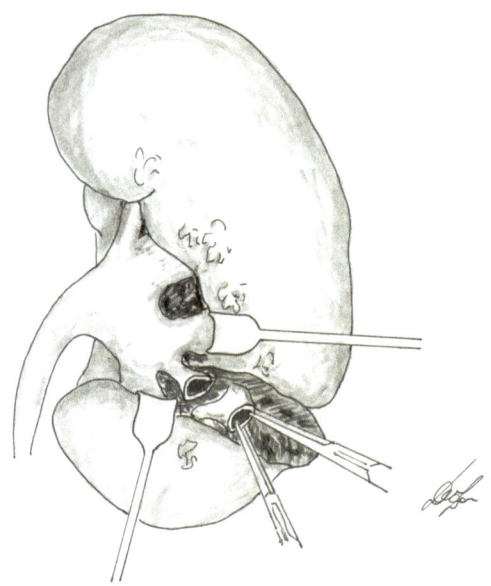

FIGURE 7.4 Lower pole lobectomy

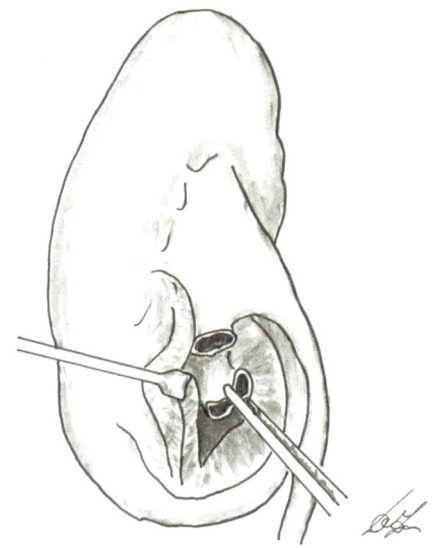

FIGURE 7.5 Lower pole lobectomy with open lower pole

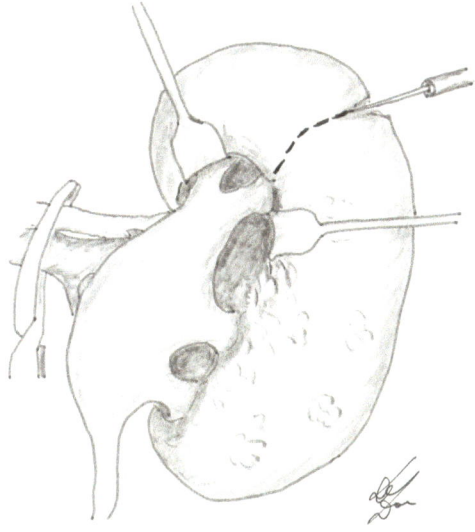

FIGURE 7.6 Upper pole nephrotomy to preparation of calyces

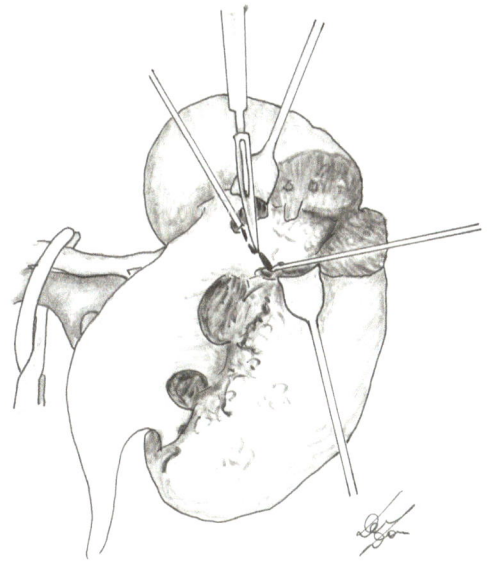

FIGURE 7.7 Upper pole lobectomy

Whatever method one chooses, renal cooling must be performed to maintain the medullary at a temperature of about 20 °C.

In cases of ischemic surgery, slow declamping promotes the vision of the bleeding source and a consequently easier hemostasis. However, clamping and declamping repeatedly is strongly to be avoided so as not to subject the kidney to subsequent reperfusion injury. The reperfusion is more dangerous than the ischemia on the renal parenchyma.

A hemostatic sponge can be placed between the surfaces, which must be approached and joined together through a continued capsular or interrupted suture.

This is the surgical outline of lobectomy or calycectomy, or renal segmentectomy. So it is clear that an important step in this type of surgery is the renal sinus opening to enter the kidney. This in fact constitutes intrarenal surgery.

7.2   Renal Sinus Access

Whenever one or more lobes are to be taken away it is critical that the renal sinus is accessed correctly. The morphology and amplitude of the renal sinus varies from individual to individual. As classically described by Henle (1866), the renal sinus is a cavity, isolated from the retroperitoneum, closed in practice and roughly rectangular in shape (5 cm high, 3 cm wide, and 2 cm deep), back to front. It is provided with two prolongations, one superior and the other inferior, which contain the major calyces.

The renal capsule is inside the sinus, in a certain sense papering the walls, thinning, and continuing with the calyceal adventitia. In this way each prolongation is lined by the kidney's internal sheet of fibrous capsule. The size and morphology of the sinus are quite variable. The cavity occupies the space from the medullar parenchyma as the external edge, and hilus as the internal edge. The hilar size and shape are also quite variable. They can be small, large, semicircular, fessuriform, even punctiform, in renal malformations. Obviously the larger the hilum is, the easier access proves to be. Its anterior lip is less expanded than the rear one, which is protruding more medially. The sinus is elastic thanks to fatty tissue that is rather abundant surround the pelvis, calyces, vessels, and nerves. The elasticity allows them to expand and retract according to their function, filling, emptying, or contracting the pelvis and calyces, and contracting or relaxing vessels. Relaxation and contraction obviously occur according to the normal or the pathological processes within the sinus cavity.

The renal capsule reaches the extrarenal pelvis and extends a thin layer of dense fibers like a sheet, which surround and adhere to the extrarenal pelvis. This sheet, already mentioned by Disse (1891) as a capsular diaphragm, totally encloses the sinus, isolating it from the retroperitoneum (Fig. 7.8). In sinusal fat there are some stringy filaments run-

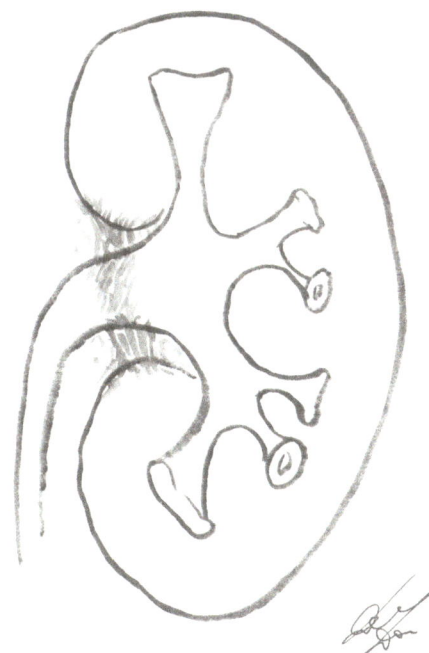

FIGURE 7.8 Disse enclosure of the renal sinus

ning from the outside of blood vessels to the pelvis, as well as the major and minor calyces. In agreement with Gil-Vernet (1984), in kidneys with sinusal sclerolipomatosis it is possible to isolate sinusal structures without damaging them, thanks to the capsular coating that divides them from the nearby sclerotic tissue.

Access to the normal renal sinus is quite easy (Figs 7.9 and 7.10). The surgical steps are as follows: (1) Blunt separation and traction towards the parenchyma of the peripyelic fat, starting at the uretero-pyelic level and proceeding up from

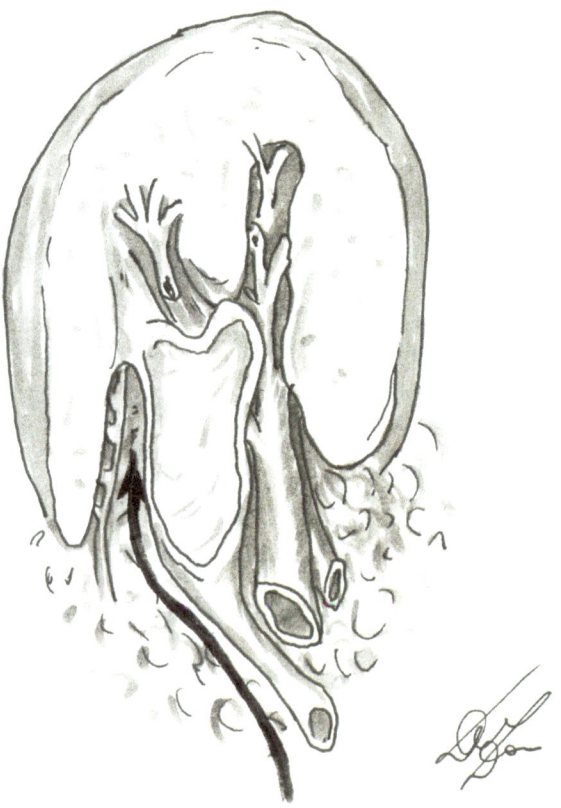

FIGURE 7.9 How to enter the renal sinus (according to G. Vernet)

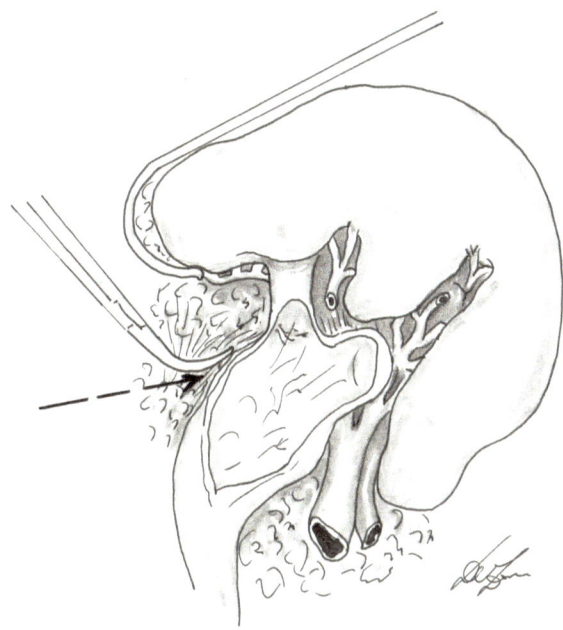

FIGURE 7.10 Pulling up the posterior polar lip facilitates the view of the minor calyx (according to G. Vernet)

there. In this way the pyelic adventitia is left separated from the fat. (2) Putting the tip of a blunt pair of scissors, kept closed, below the capsular diaphragm, closing the pyelic adventitia then sharply opening it in order to achieve a generally rare capsular resistance. (3) Open the sinus entrance and once inside the sinus, an *ad hoc* handled retractor is placed, retaining the whole mass of peripyelic fat, capsule, the internal lip of the posterior renal edge, and the retropyelic vessels. The access is from the renal posterior face and it is easy to retract the block of tissue upwards without damaging or tearing the parenchyma, since, protected by a capsule and by usually dense peripyelic fat, it has great resistance and elasticity. The endosinusal structures are now visible. (4) By pushing gently, as deep as possible, an open wet gauze completes the dissection without bleeding. (5) In the posterior access, once the gauze is removed, the parenchymal lip is pulled with a second retractor, which closes the sinus.

The same process is followed for anterior access: the sinus concavity is more pronounced and open given the lateral rim retraction compared to the posterior one. For that reason, only considering the sinus entrance, access seems more facilitated, but to identify the pelvis and calyces it is necessary to separate the vessels, artery/ies and vein/s, from the pelvis. This represents a delicate surgical moment and a consequent risk, since the vessels must be moved from the pyelo-calyceal structures. For that reason the posterior side is generally chosen.

The aforementioned procedure assumes that the sinus is in a normal state. Stones, particularly those in the mould or staghorns, many types of inflammation, and malformative pathologies could greatly alter the hilum and sinus anatomy through a perirenal, peripyelic, and endorenal reaction, which is sometimes very severe, creating a more complicated, though not impossible, sinus access.

The author is in complete agreement with Gill-Vernet's description: "...the most advisable procedure is to identify the most superior and free part of the ureter and from there follow a retrograde dissection with blunt-end scissors through the sclerolipomatous mass following a detachment plan which is always present between the pyelic adventitia and the peripyelitis. It is advisable to free the posterior surface of the pelvis from the sclerosed shell that enwraps it."

Commonly, the innersinusal sclero-lipomatosis is less intense than the outersinusal one and that of the peripyelo-ureteric varices. This forms the basis for a guide to the surgical technique that starts far from the hilum, distally, at the level of a normal ureter and well distal to the sclerolipomatosis, where there is no pyelo-ureteritis.

The important thing to note in surgery of this kind is never to leave the adventitial plane of the ureter and pelvis. Into this plane place the tip of a closed blunt pair of scissors and push it gently upwards, close to the adventitia until it reaches the peripyelitis, i.e. sclerosis and sclerolipomatosis. There is always a thin space between the adventitia and fat sclerosis. With great care and patience continue to push the closed scissors as far as possible. The fat must be cut and opened but not removed, since the presence of the fat in the peripyelic vessels is usually not visible due to the sclerosis. The scissors should now be between the peripyelic fat and the pyelic adventitia, where there is always a plane along which one can run the blunt scissors. This is a guideline that must always be borne in mind (Figs. 7.11, 7.12, 7.13, and 7.14).

According to the amplitude and shape of the pyelo-ureteric junction, of the pelvis, and of their inflammatory coverage, it could be necessary to open the sclerosis with a

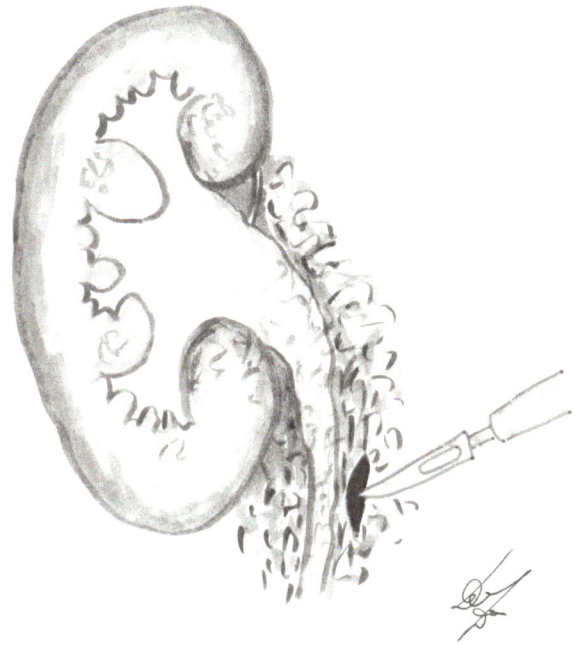

FIGURE 7.11 In difficult conditions, like pyelo-calycal sclerolipomatosis, it is always possible to enter the sinus since there is a space between the excretory ducts adventitia and the sclerotic tissue. Under normal conditions it is usual to start from the ureter (according to G. Vernet)

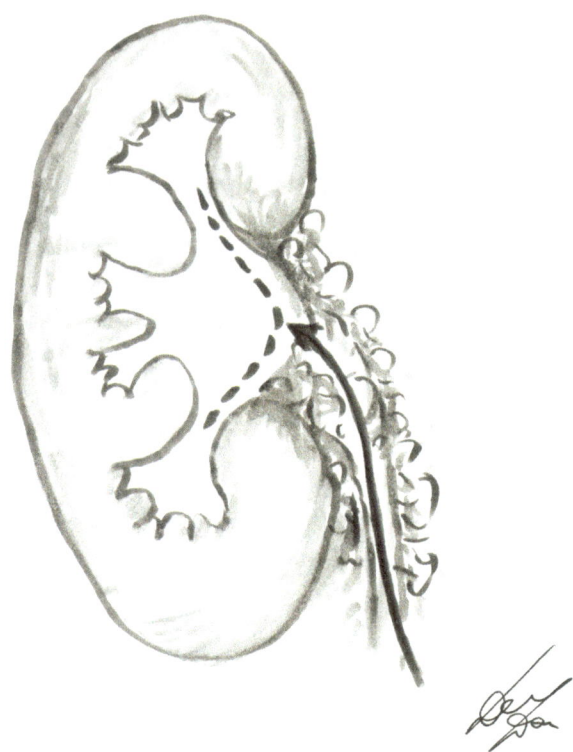

FIGURE 7.12 How to reach the sinus

little cut, which will gradually set the ureter and the pelvis free. It is extremely important to leave the adventitia sound.

The fat must be opened and accurately dissected from the pelvis, but not removed, since it covers peripyelic vessels, often not visible because of the thickness of the multiple sclerosis. Liberation of the intrasinusal structures will result in an emergency situation in the major calyces. Careful dissection will facilitate prudent freeing of all tougher fat and renal parenchyma. Once the major calyx has been visualized, a

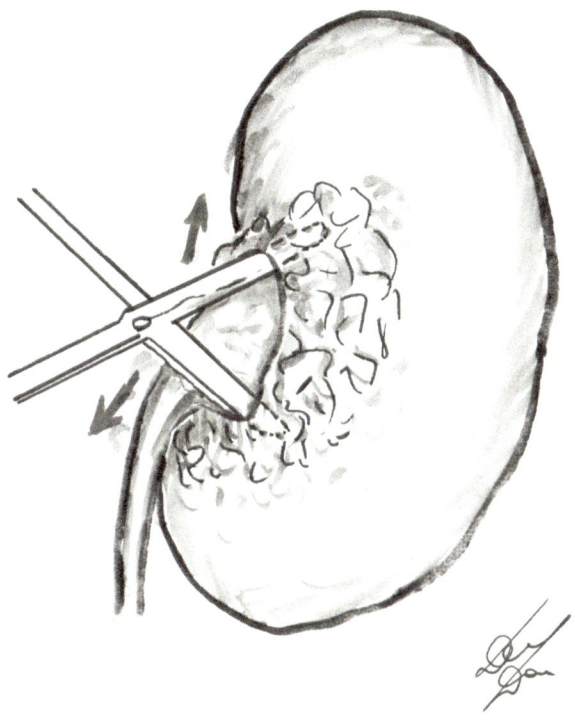

Figure 7.13 A gentle push with a blunt-closed pair of scissors creates a space between sclerotic and normal tissue. A small cut on the pathologic area and vigorous opening of the scissors amplify the space (according to G. Vernet)

more vigorous freeing of sclerotic tissue and the sinusal parenchyma covering it will isolate the minor calyces without producing any harm. Deep gentle pushing of a soaked gauze will help isolate the intrarenal structures between the adventitia and reactive tissue, and reveal the minor calyx without creating damage.

The next part of the operation will be done accord to the lesions present.

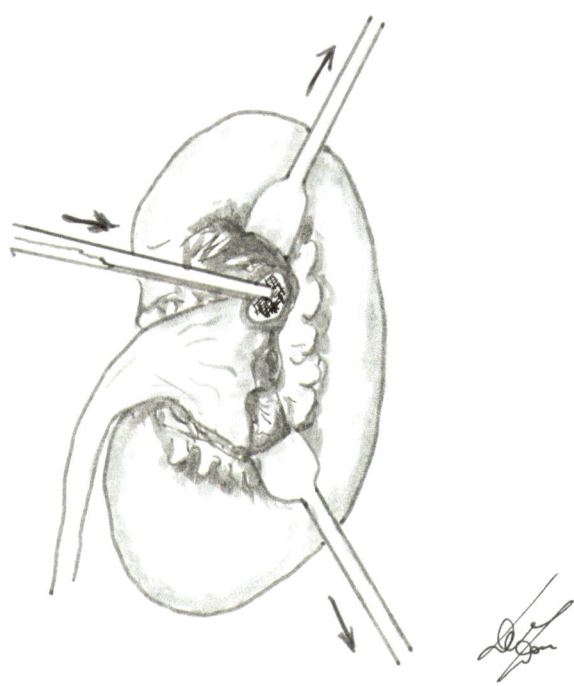

FIGURE 7.14 A gentle push with a wet gauze or a sponge promotes entry into the deep sinus at the level of the calyco-pyramidal junction (according to G. Vernet)

7.3   Pathologic Situations Potentially Requiring Endosinusal Access

Undoubtedly the conditions that could necessitate endosinusal access to the intrarenal collecting system are not frequent occurrences. They include calyx or pyelic substance loss, their stenosis, malformations (such cysts, diverticula), localized and removable neoplasms, vascular pathologies interfering with calyco-pyelic dynamics, and the presence of stones that, due to their shape and dimensions need intrarenal surgery. Consequenty, pyelo-calycolithotomies, calyceal resections, end-to-end calyceal sutures, calycoplastics, calycopyeloplastics, bipolar calycocalycostomies, pyelocalycoplastics, and capsulopyeloplastics represent surgical techniques capable of curing or treating those pathologic conditions that utilize wide access to the renal sinus after hilum dissection.

Among those techniques that require ample opening of the renal sinus, one is of particular interest for the topic we are discussing: segmental resection or renal segmentectomy.

7.4   Renal Segmental Resection (Lobectomy, Calycectomy, Segmentectomy)

Renal segmental resection, also known as a calycectomy or, rather, a calyx-based resection, is the removal of a renal lobe (lobectomy) individualized through a minor calyx. It includes the pyramid apex, which is surrounded by cortical tissue like a cup. As mentioned in the introduction, with this kind of resection the residual parenchyma, in which the removed lobe (or lobes) had its natural parenchymal, vascular, and nervous individuality, is left sound.

Typical indications for this type of operation include pyelo-calyceal stones together with the resulting regional complication of pyelonephritis localized in one or more lobes, due to minor or medium calculolytic calyx clogging. In such cases simple stone removal allows for stone relapses in the very diseased parenchyma. However, segmental resection in such circumstances abolishes the cause of the disease, the stone, the effects of this on the parenchyma, the pyelonephritis, and the basis for stone recurrence, leaving the residual parenchyma completely sound and healthy.

In case of persistent surgical indications, the same can be said for hydronephrosis that is localized in one area and caused by an obstruction of a calyx tributary in a part of the hydronephrotic parenchyma, which is not further reparable and is caused by the calyceal obstruction, while the remainder of the kidney is normal.

Another example could be pyelocalyceal stenosis amendable with calycopyeloplastics. In this instance (Figs. 7.15, 7.16,

7.17, 7.18, 7.19, and 7.20) the inferior small calyx restores the
normality of the pyelic cavity. The calyx is isolated at a polar
level, detached from the apex papillae, opened, spatulated,
and overturned on the breach of the pelvis and opened
beyond the stenosis narrowing. The ablation of the lobe without its own calyx is not a true privation of normal tissue, since
the stenosis certainly had an effect on the parenchyma, as
hydronephrosis is to be expected after a calyceal stenosis.
Thus a lobectomy following calycopyeloplastic surgery is
curative in every sense.

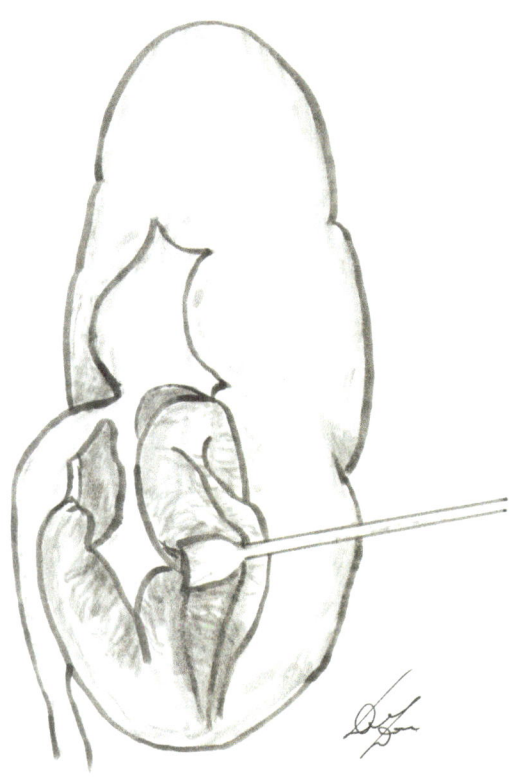

FIGURE 7.15 Calico-pyeloplastic surgery: the pelvis stricture is
resolved through a wide pyelo-calical incision (personal technique)

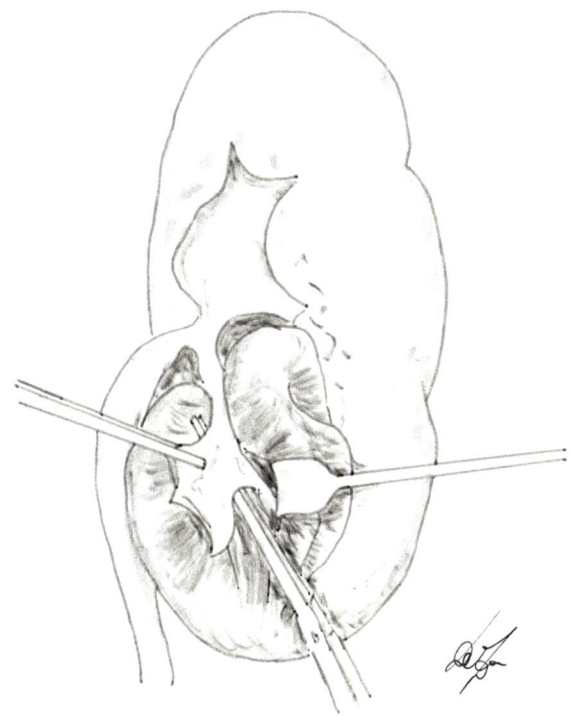

FIGURE 7.16 Calico-pyeloplastic surgery: calyceal preparation and dissection of the calyx

These are examples of infrequent pathologic conditions. As has been mentioned several times, the indications for renal segmentectomies are quite rare because the pathologies that potentially require that kind of surgery are rare themselves. However, rare does not means non-existent!

When there is an indication for surgery, the technique, despite its rarity, allows you to save the kidney and to occasionally treat very severe conditions.

Below is a descriptions of a typical inferior calycectomy or lobectomy.

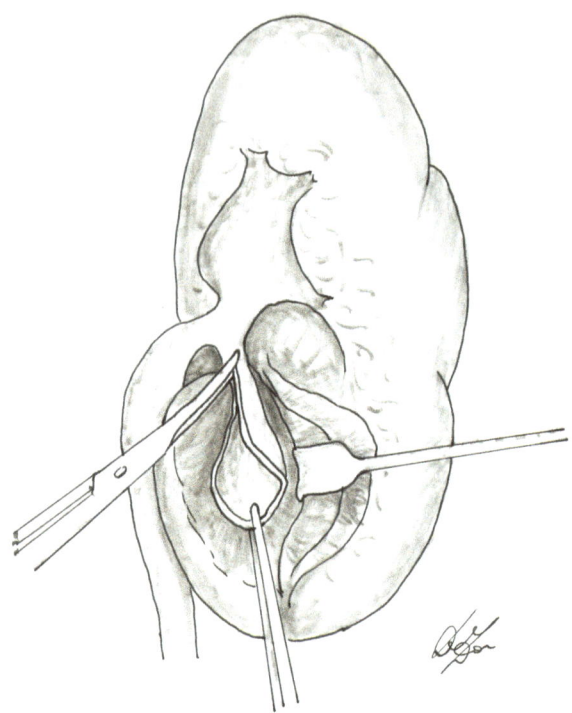

FIGURE 7.17 Calico-pyeloplastic surgery: calico-pyramid amputation and calyceal spatulation

In open surgery, the kidney is reached via an oblique, anterior access, such as a Fey incision. The peritoneum is detached using a smooth, blunt dissection from the Gerota fascia. After that a deep dissection will reach the ureter, which will be freed as far as the pelvis, once the renal lodge has been opened. The kidney is isolated from the anterior and posterior fasciae and the posterior surface is exposed. The renal sinus is freed from the Disse capsular closure, thus opening the sinus entrance. As described above, once inside the sinus,

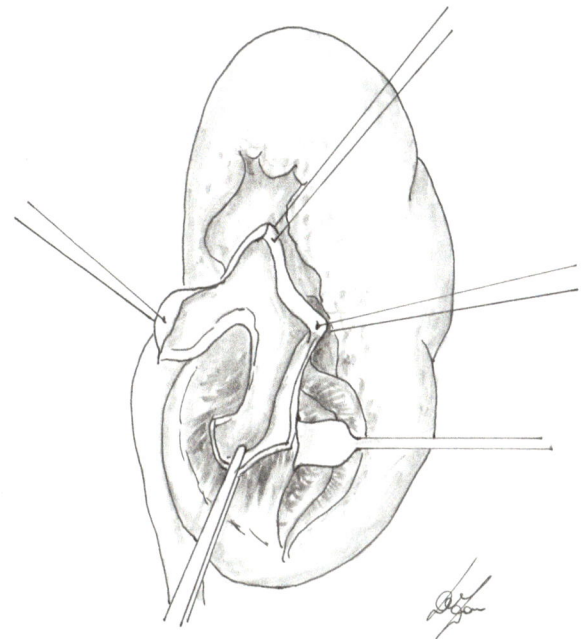

FIGURE 7.18 Calico-pyeloplastic surgery: overturning of the spatulated calyceal flap

the major calyces are identified thanks to the delicate traction of the parenchyma and endorenal fat: a small nephrotomy is done in the direction of the small calyx that needs to be reached. The traction on the lips of the cut parenchyma produces the hemostasis of the ordinarily unimportant bleeding. The minor calyx is followed until it reaches the apex papillae. The anatomic situation will guide the progressive parenchymal cut so far that it will be possible to follow the anterior, posterior, and lateral edges of the desired lobe we have identified through a gentle traction on the calyx (Figs. 7.4, 7.5, 7.6, and 7.7).

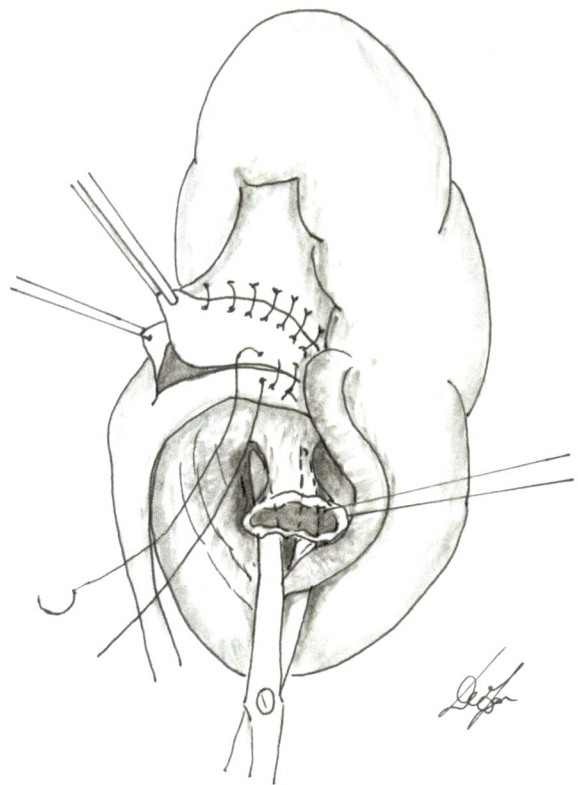

FIGURE 7.19 Calico-pyeloplastic surgery: adjusting and suturing the calical flap on the opened pelvis and tributary parenchymal resection

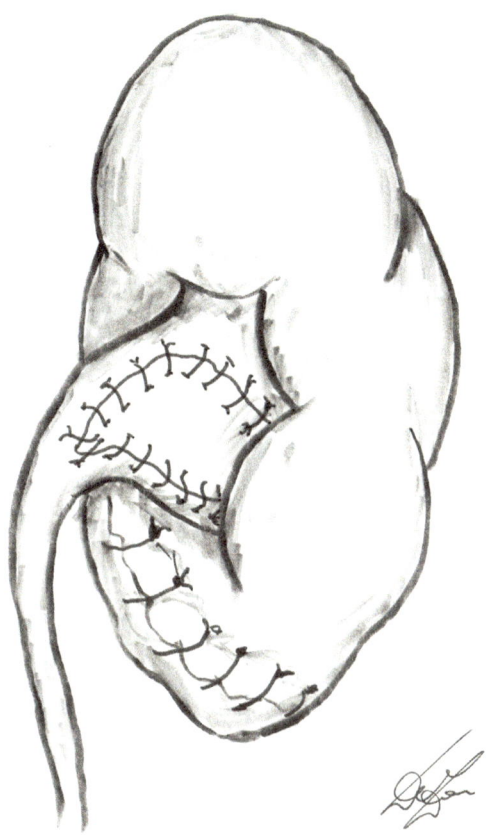

FIGURE 7.20 Calico-pyeloplastic surgery: removing the damaged, hydronephrotic lobe through a typical lobectomy

7.5   Reconstructive Surgery of the Intrarenal Collecting System

Endorenal plastic surgery is not common, but the pathologic conditions that necessitate it are less rare than one may assume. As far as excretory endorenal pathway alterations are concerned, endoscopic, minimally invasive techniques have certainly led to an improvement in post-instrumental outcomes compared to the post-surgical ones. This has also been explained by the fact that they are better received by

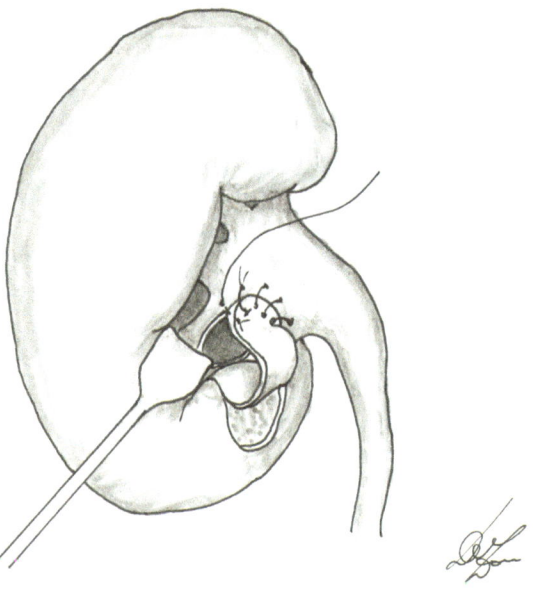

FIGURE 7.21 Capsulo-calicoplasty for small lower calyx defect

patients and, as a result, they are implemented at an earlier stage compared to open surgery. The absence of delays in treatment plays an important role in the post-instrumental integrity of the excretory pathway. Nevertheless, despite being infrequent, injuries and renal function disorders may exist. When this is the case knowing such problems exist is important in order to implement the correct treatment.

Some lesions are mendable endoscopically or through minor operations, others instead require more delicate, complex surgery (Figs. 7.21, 7.22, 7.23, 7.24, and 7.25). In any case a wide sinus opening will be necessary.

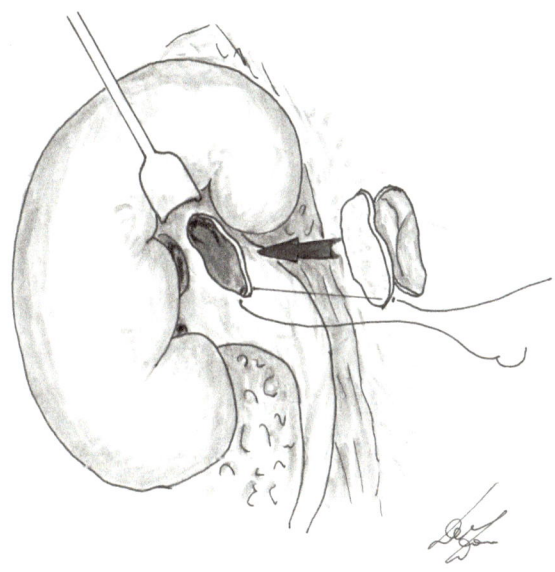

Figure 7.22 Peritoneo-calicoplasty for small upper calix defect

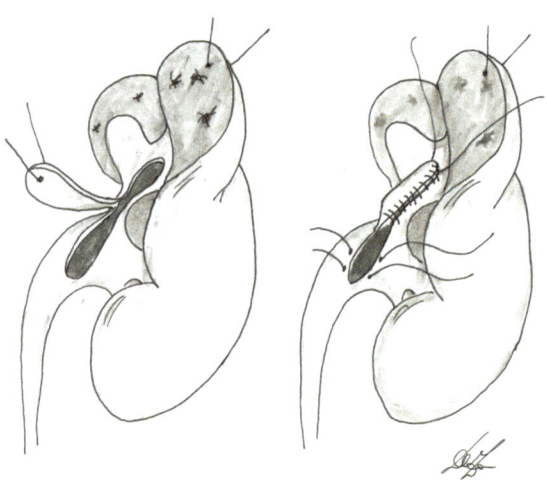

FIGURE 7.23 Pyelo-calicoplastic surgery: reversed Culp operation, only possible when there is a large pelvis (personal technique)

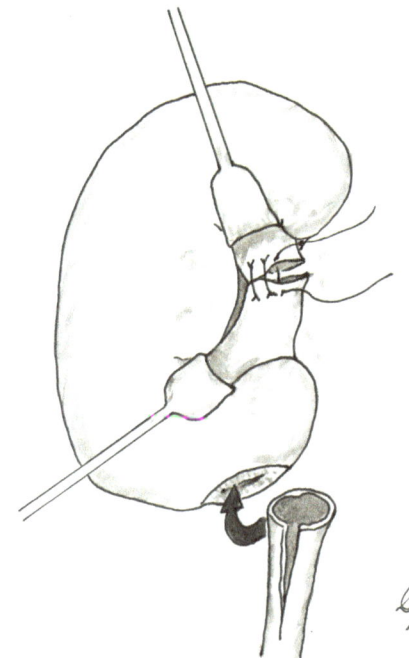

FIGURE 7.24 Pelvis ablation, bipolar calico-calicostomy and spatulated uretero-polarcali-costomy. Smith operation: see text

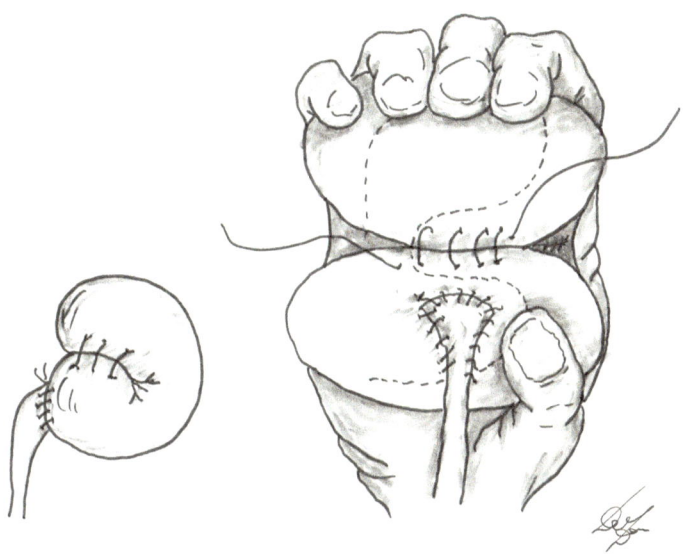

FIGURE 7.25 Hand hydronephrotic compression in the Smith operation: see text

7.6 Calyceal Stenosis

Minor or major calyceal stenosis, if treated early, can be solved endoscopically through a targeted calycotomy with or without endoscopic or percutaneous intubation. If only recognized belatedly and then associated with districtual hydronephrosis and pericalyceal sclerosis they require a uni- or plurilobar segmentectomy, depending on the size of the stenosis on the minor or major calyx. If recognized at a stage that is neither particularly early or late, the restricted zone resection and end-to-end suturing could, in theory, be practiced, provided there is no large pericalyceal sclerosis. A wide renal sinus opening is necessary to correctly identify the calyx and the stenosis extension, thus determining the length of the nephrotomy needed.

Once stenosis and its extension have been individualized and the presence or absence of peristenosis sclerotic deep-

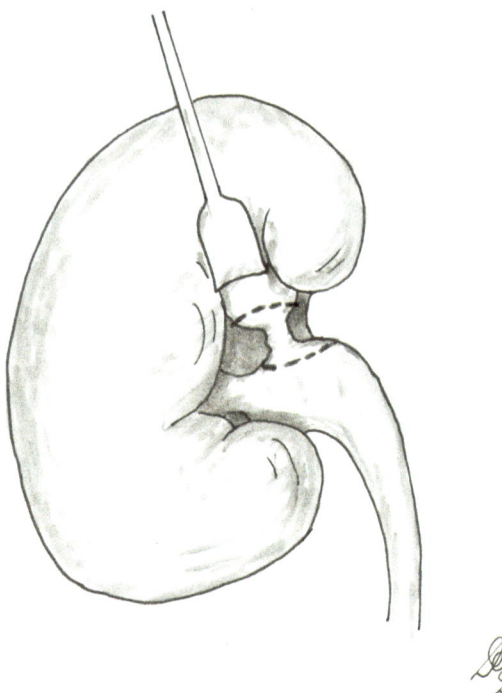

FIGURE 7.26 Calyceal stenosis

ness has been demonstrated, and if calyceal resection and end-to-end suture seem possible, the following operation will be made, as shown in Figs. 7.26 and 7.27. The calyceal wall suture must be completely tensionless. However, such circumstances also apply in the indications for a simple stenosis incision and intubation. Thus, the calyceal resection remains the preferred choice compared to an easier operation. Indications for segmentectomy are, however, exceptional.

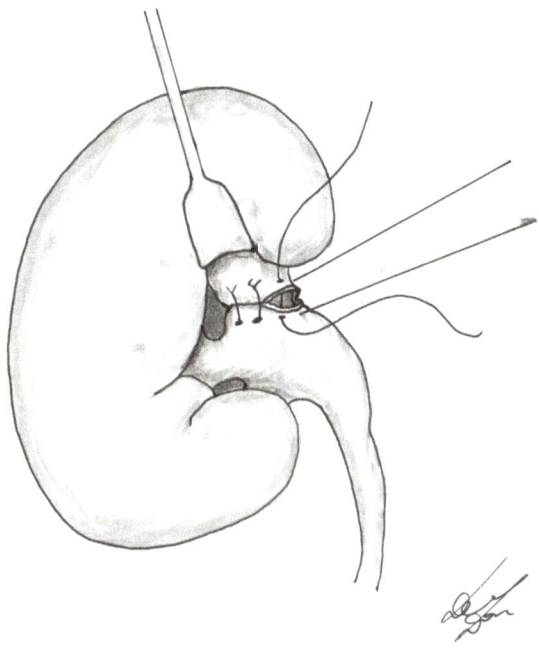

FIGURE 7.27 Calyceal stenosis: end-to-end suture after calyceal resection for stenosis; rear view

7.7 Pyelic, Pyelo-Calyceal Stenosis, or Coarctation

Pyelic stenosis and pyelic coarctation are commonly the results of long-standing stones or of many poorly managed surgeries. They are not frequent and neither is pyelocaliceal stenosis. When present, they create a type of parenchymal harm that is serious due to duct dilation or interstitial sclerosis. Their correction requires calycopyeloplastic surgery similar to that described by the author in 1979 and previously shown in Figs. 7.15, 7.16,

7.17, 7.18, 7.19, and 7.20). The operation starts with the isolation of the pelvis and major calyx in the renal sinus through a small nephrotomy in the direction of the minor sloping calyx, if inferior, and of the upward sloping one if superior, reaching the apex of the papilla. Ample calicopyelotomy must overtake and exceed the stenosis. Amputate the calyx, detaching it from the papilla. Control the wide spatulation of the detached calyx overtaking and exceeding the coarctation zone before reaching the normal tissue. Isolate the open calyx from each side to mobilize and overturn it on the wide opening obtained using spatulation. Suture the margins of the overturned calyx to those of the calicopyelotomy, achieving a width corresponding to that of the chosen calyx. In the case of more serious coarctation it may be necessary to use the width of a bigger calyx. Obviously a lobe or lobes without calyceal discharge have to be removed. From there the operation continues with a typical segmentectomy.

The damage incurred to the kidney is practically nonexistent because the removed parenchyma was not sound, as it was harmed by coartaction and the consequent flogistic and hydronephrotic consequences.

7.8   Calyceal Prolonged Stenosis

This is the case with the superior calyx, since it is the longest. The prolonged stenosis may be repaired in some cases by using a technique that was successfully experimented with by the author: in practice it is like the procedure described by Culp [194] for correction of the pyelo-ureteric fault, only inverted. It is not a pyelo-ureteric but pyelocalyceal plastic surgery. As the reader knows, Culp [194] suggested for the pyelo-ureteric joint enlargement using a plastic operation, consisting of taking an oblique pelvic strip, with an inferior base. The pelvic incision for the strip was prolonged through the open joint on the ureter for a couple of centimeters. The peduncle base then bordered the opened joint and ureter. The flap was then rotated and turned down so as to cover the hole of the open joint and ureter. The flap and ureter margins were sutured with the desired result of widening the joint that was previously narrowed.

The pyelo-ureteric faults are similar to those of the superior calyx in that a positive result from the surgical technique relies upon a large pelvis, all the better if it is abundant.

The technique described by the author [195] is as follows: widen the opening of the anterior or posterior renal sinus, according to the depth of the calyx inside the parenchyma, preoperatively demonstrated by imaging and endoscopic examinations. Once the superior calyx has been reached it emerges from the pelvis. The execution of this part of the technique into the sinus must be performed as carefully as possible. A nephrotomy above the calyx is made as long as the length of the shrinkage, which is now visible. A frank incision of the stenosis must be performed according to the length and width of the area that is covered. Next is the creation of an oblique flap on the exposed pelvis' pedunculated anterior surface, which borders the calyceal part that was previously opened using a long incision beyond the stenosis. The flap on the widely opened superior stenotic calyx is rotated. Obviously the length and width of the flap must perfectly correspond to those that are to be covered in order to obtain the desired calyceal caliber normalization. The overlapped flap and calicotomy margins are sutured. There is no suture tension, provided that the length of the area to be covered and flap measures were correct (Fig. 7.23).

A small pelvis, like those of early calyces branching, are not suited to this kind of plastic surgery.

7.9   Pelvis Ablation

There are exceptional situations in which pathologies that are strictly localized in the renal pelvis and that involve all pelvic tissue practically prevent it from functioning. This includes renal function. This is often caused by the inauspicious results of repeated endoscopic or open surgical operations.

It may be necessary, in such cases, to remove the irreparably damaged pelvis because of the absence of sound, utilizable tissue or because of its intrinsic pathology. On the other hand, the calyces may be normal, although very dilated as is (normal) with the ureter. In those cases a large hydronephrosis is present due to the pathologic noxa that caused the dilation of the calyces that were still naturally healthy. In spite of the severe hydronephrosis, the kidney could still be capable of working well enough and its chemo-physical function must be preserved as in the case of a solitary kidney. It is then necessary to choose between nephrectomy and dialysis in the case of a solitary kidney and pelvectomy with calico-ureteric patency reconstruction.

The pelvic ablation that follows the wide opening of the renal sinus and the visualization of major calyces does not pose any problems whatsoever, with the exception of the pelvis liberation by present peripyelitis, which can be very intense. The situation after pelvectomy involves strongly dilated major calyces, remarkable hydronephrosis, and a normal ureter. When possible the calicostomy is performed inside the sinus terminally between the two infundibula or laterally after closing the pyelo-calyceal mouths. The closure must be done through a perfect suture. The ureter will be 1 cm spatulated. The anastomosis between the opened ureter and the polar hydronephrotic cavity is quite easy to perform since the calycectasis practically reaches the renal capsule. The spatulation of the ureteral ending has value in obtaining a large anastomotic surface capable of a good hydronephrotic discharge. The anastomotic suture will be anchored to the renal capsule and coated (Fig. 7.24).

In order to facilitate the calyceal anastomosis, it is possible to bring the two poles close together through manual compression, given the poor renal consistency that arises as a result of the serious hydronephrosis shown in Fig. 7.25.

It goes without saying that those operations, first described by Hamilton Stewart in 1957, and subsequently performed by Smith, Dunn, and Roberts in 1979 [197–199], are extremely rare.

7.10   Open, Laparoscopic, Robotic Surgery

The delicacy, complexity, and difficulty of the operations described assume that classic surgery, namely open, is compulsory. The literature review of the topic shows that laparoscopic and robotic surgery are available with good results for renal resections and intrarenal operations. At present I am yet to see typical segmentectomies executed in this way, but I have no doubt that, when the indications are correct, segmentectomies will be done via laparoscopy and robotics [200–210].

Not being expert in those techniques myself I felt it necessary to ask my friends and experienced colleagues to offer their results on intrasinusal surgery and possibly on intrarenal collecting system operations.

Prof. Muto, Head of the Urology Department at the Campus Medical University, Rome, sent me clear photographs of intrarenal laparoscopic surgery for pelvic and calyceal stones (Figs. 7.28, 7.29, 7.30, 7.31, 7.32, and 7.33). Looking

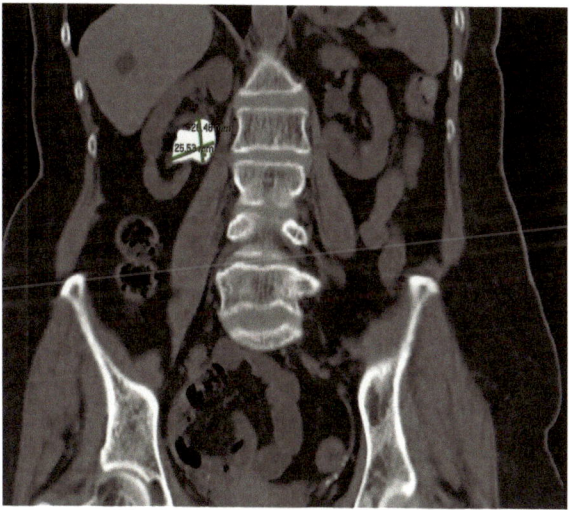

Figure 7.28 Coronaric RM section. Large, stag-horn stone of the right kidney, occupying the pelvis and major calyces (courtesy of Prof. G. Muto)

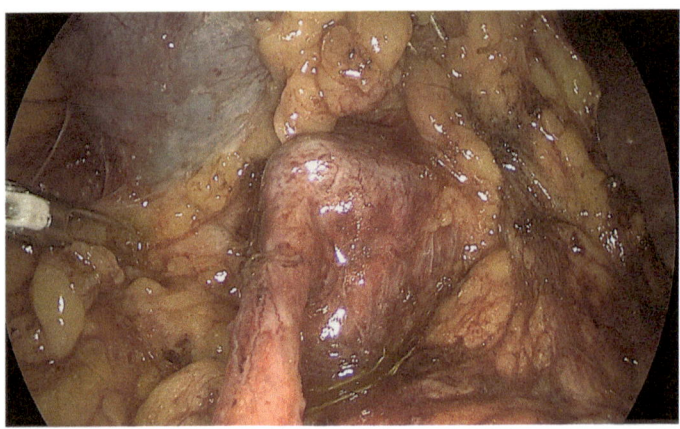

FIGURE 7.29 Laparoscopy, intrarenal large exposure of the intra-sinusal area and pelvis and calyces individualization. Intraoperative photo (courtesy of Prof. G. Muto)

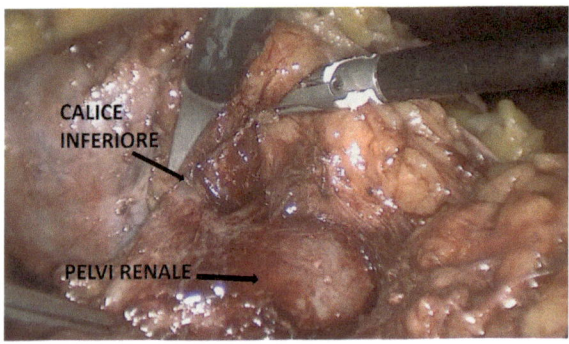

FIGURE 7.30 Laparoscopy, intrarenal large exposure of the intrasinusal area and pelvis and calyces individualization: inferior calyx preparation. Intraoperative laparoscopic photo (courtesy of Prof. G. Muto)

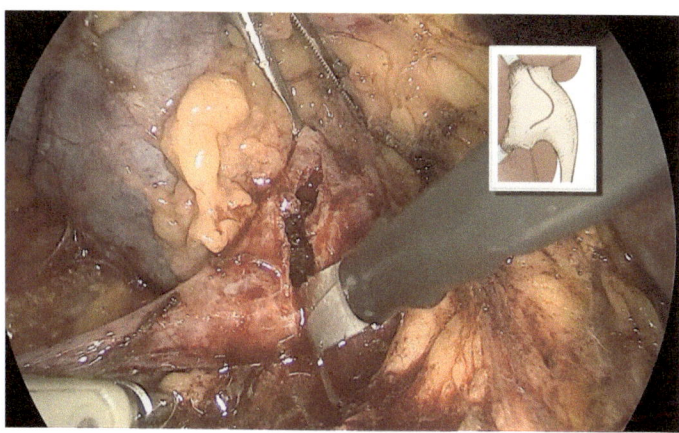

FIGURE 7.31 Laparoscopy, intrarenal large exposure of the intra-sinusal area and pelvis and calyces individualization: large opening of the pelvis and calyces with a Gil Vernet incision. Intraoperative laparoscopic photo (courtesy of Prof. G. Muto)

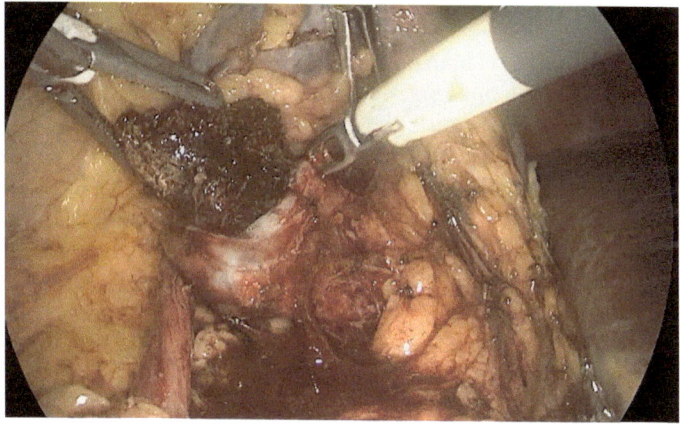

FIGURE 7.32 Laparoscopy, intrarenal large exposure of the intra-sinusal area and pelvis and calyces individualization: moving the stone. Intraoperative laparoscopic photo (courtesy of Prof. G. Muto)

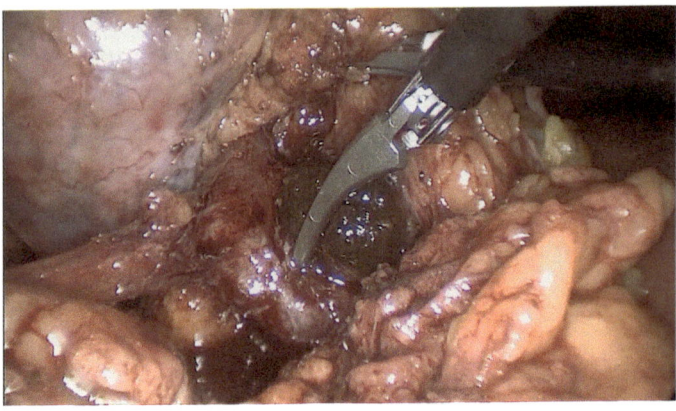

FIGURE 7.33 Laparoscopy, intrarenal large exposure of the intra-sinusal area and pelvis and calyces individualization: removing the stone. Intraoperative laparoscopic photo (courtesy of Prof. G. Muto)

at the images it easy to understand how wide the renal sinus opening was and how the intrarenal pelvic and calyceal preparation was clean enough to perform a Gil Vernet calico-pyelo-calyceal opening. The intrarenal elements thus completely dominate inside the sinus.

Prof. Muto also informs us that, considering the choice among various mini-invasive techniques used to remove stones from the kidney, the European Guidelines suggest that laparoscopy is used only for complex stones, more than 2 cm in extrarenal pelvis, or in cases of endoscopic failures, or in stones with associated pyelo-ureteric joint pathology. Prof. Muto also cites the same relatively recent papers in which 60 patients were divided into two groups, the first group for endoscopic treatment and the second for laparoscopic treatment. The second group of patients had less bleeding, less need for transfusion, and less decrease in renal function. Other authors, according to Prof. Muto, affirm that laparoscopic treatment, compared with endoscopic treatment, has a lower failure percentage, less bleeding, less need for transfusion, and less septic complications, but more stone free rate.

Prof. Porpiglia, Head of the Urology Department at Tourin University, San Luigi d'Orbassano Hospital, kindly sent me some clear photographs of two laparoscopic operations of cali-cectomies, one for a hydrocalyx with multiple stones and the second for a Fraley syndrome (Figs. 7.34 and 7.35). As he told me several times, robotics and laparoscopy are able to perform intrarenal surgery and collecting system operations the same as in open surgery and the cases presented are cases in point.

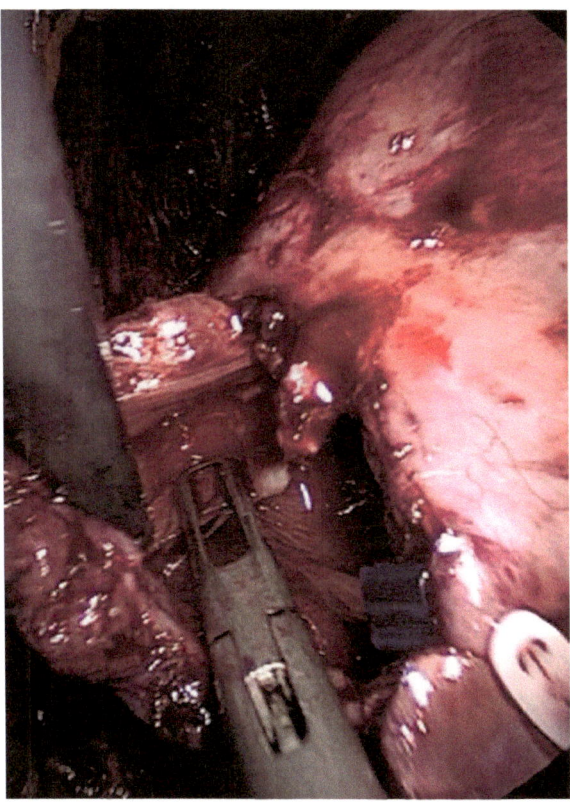

FIGURE 7.34 Hydrocalyx in the right kidney with multiple stones at the CT scan. Intraoperative photo from outside the nephrotomy and smooth dissection of the calyceal mucosa (courtesy of Prof. F. Porpiglia)

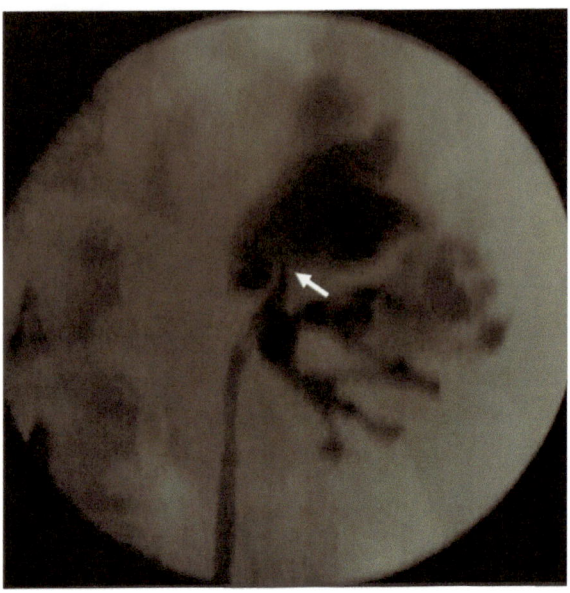

FIGURE 7.35 Abdominal CT scan suggests the presence of a crossing vessel at the *left upper* pole infundibulum, resulting in a hydronephrosis (courtesy of Prof. F. Porpiglia)

Medical records of the first case consisted of a hydrocalyx with multiple stones: "45-year-old patient affected by moderate right flank pain for some years." Abdominal US showed evidence of right kidney calyx dilatation with some stones inside. CT scan confirmed the dilatation of middle right renal calyx with multiple stones. The patient was scheduled for a laparoscopic calicectomy. A retroperitoneoscopic approach was chosen. The kidney was exposed opening the renal fascia from the lateral margin. A nephrotomy was performed in the mesorenal region to reach the calyx. The calyx was opened and the stones removed. The calyx mucosa was then dissected from the renal parenchyma. A delicate suture was performed to close the calyceal infundibulum. Finally, the kidney was sutured at the level of a nephrotomy. No operative or postoperative complications were recorded" (Figs. 7.34, 7.36, 7.37, 7.38, and 7.39).

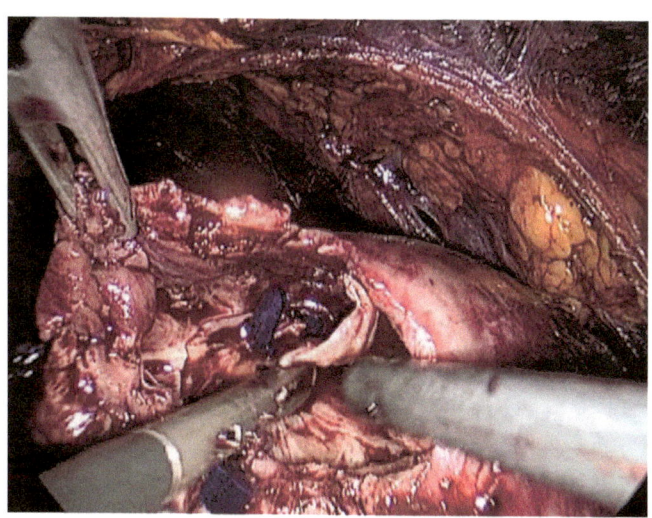

FIGURE 7.36 Hydrocalyx in the right kidney with multiple stones shown on the CT scan: nephrotomy and preparating the opened calyx. Intraoperative laparoscopic photo (courtesy of Prof. F. Porpiglia)

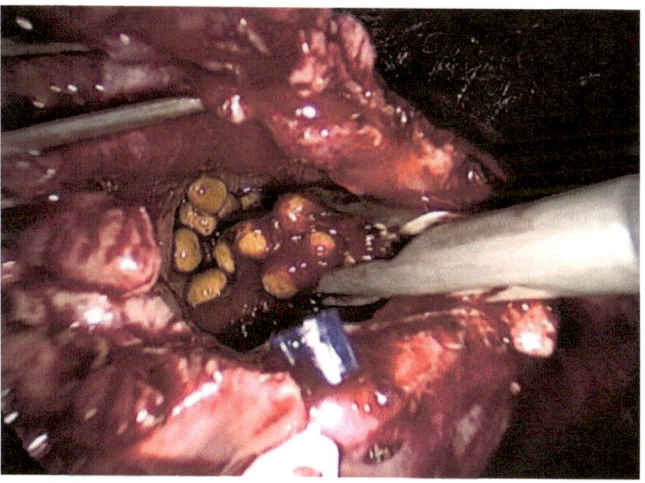

FIGURE 7.37 Hydrocalyx in the right kidney with multiple stones shown on the CT scan: stone removal. Intraoperative laparoscopic photo (courtesy of Prof. F. Porpiglia)

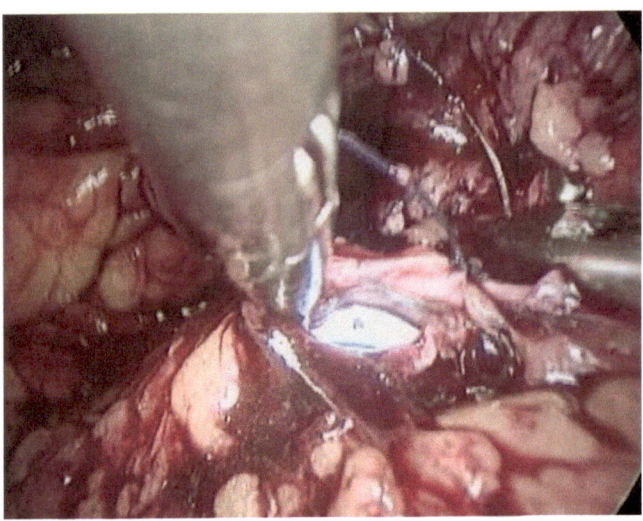

FIGURE 7.38 Hydrocalyx in the right kidney with multiple stones shown on the CT scan: preparation for the suture. Intraoperative laparoscopic photo (courtesy of Prof. F. Porpiglia)

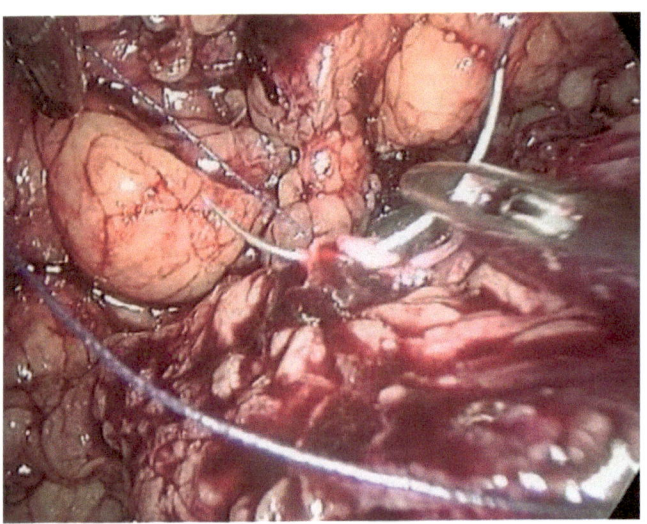

FIGURE 7.39 Hydrocalyx in the right kidney with multiple stones shown on the CT scan: suture of the calyceal orifice with POS 3/0 locked with Lapra-7. Intra-operative photo (courtesy of Prof. F. Porpiglia)

Medical records of the second case "Laparoscopic Nephron-Sparing Calycectomy For Fraley'S Syndrome" (Figs. 7.35, 7.40, 7.41, 7.42, 7.43, 7.44, 7.45, 7.46, and 7.47) are as follows: Young female, 46 years old. Medical history of dyslipidemia, uterine currettage, and previous miscarriage. Urological history of recurrent cystitis and pyelonephritis with left flank pain managed conservatively. Screening urinalysis detection of microscopic hematuria. Ultrasound evidence of dilatation of the left upper calyx. Abdominal CT scan suggests the possibility of a crossing vessel at the left upper pole infundibulum resulting in an hydrocalycosis. The nuclear renal scan demonstrates the tracer persistence trapped in the right upper pole calyx, although the other parts of the kidney drained promptly. At the time of surgery, a retrograde pyelogram demonstrates the upper pole calyx dilation with a filling defect corresponding to a vascular impression on the infundibulum. For the surgical treatment, a retroperitoneum laparoscopic approach is chosen. After placing the trocars, the posterior pararenal and perirenal fatty areas are dissected to gain access to the kidney. The upper pole is identified. It appears redundant due to upper calyx dilatation. Renal sinus and vascular pedicle are identified and

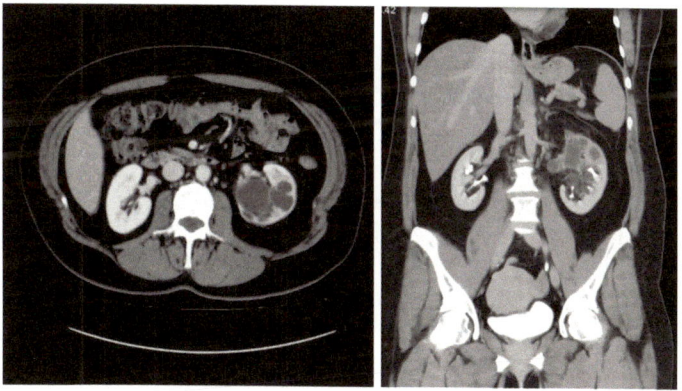

FIGURE 7.40 A vessel crossing at the left upper pole infundibulum resulting in a hydronephrosis: preoperative pyelography confirms the diagnosis (courtesy of Prof. F. Porpiglia)

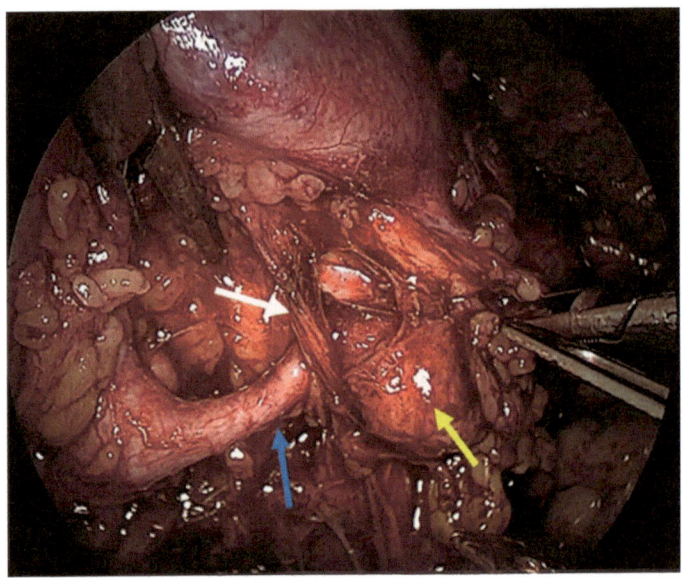

FIGURE 7.41 A vessel crossing at the left upper pole infundibulum resulting in a hydronephrosis: the renal pelvis appears normal in size, but in the upper part of the collecting system the superior calyx is dilated (*yellow arrow*) due to an obstruction generated by a segmentally crossing vessel (*white arrow*) at the level of calyceal infundibulum (*blue arrow*). Intraoperative laparoscopic photo (courtesy of Prof. F. Porpiglia)

dissected. The renal pelvis appears normal, but in the upper part of the collecting system the superior calyx is dilated due to an obstruction generated by a segmental crossing vessel at the level of the calyceal infundibulum. The crossing vessel and the upper calyceal indundibulum are not dissected. The calyceal infundibulum is clipped with reassorbable clips to avoid the risk of migration after the surgery; then it is sectioned. A smooth dissection of the calyx is performed, without any clamping of segmental branches, preserving the thin layer of renal parenchyma of the upper pole of the kidney. In the deepest phase of the calycectomy the renal papilla and

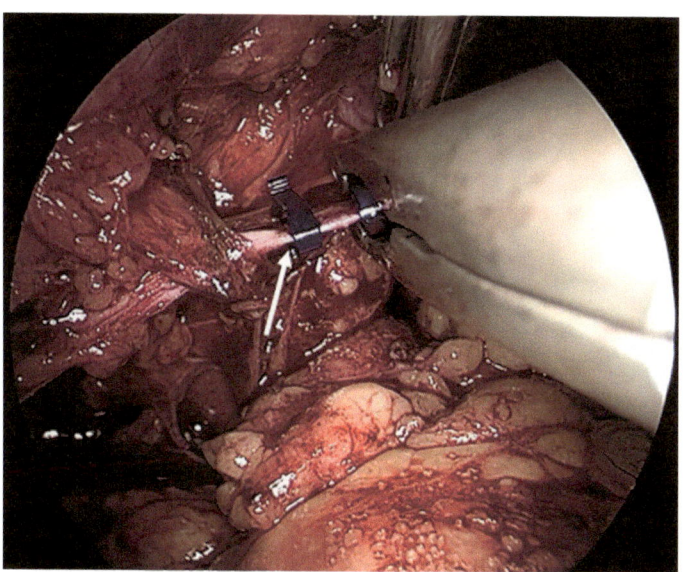

Figure 7.42 A vessel crossing at the left upper pole infundibulum resulting in a hydronephrosis: the calyceal infundibulum (*white arrow*) is clipped with reabsorbable clips to avoid the risk of migration after the surgery, then it is sectioned. Intraoperative laparoscopic photo (courtesy of Prof. F. Poroiglia)

the sinus fat are identified and the smooth muscular fibers of the anchoring calyx were dissected. The calyx is completely removed in order to avoid the risk of urinary fistulas. At the end of the extirpative phase, the upper pole sinusal cavity is examined in order to identify parenchymal structures like the renal papilla and Columns of Bertin. The interlobar vessels at this level are selectively coagulated, avoiding intrasinusal hematoma. To complete the procedure, the perirenal fat is inserted inside the cavity and fixed with PDS 2/0 in order to prevent the risk of bleeding and urinary fistulas."

Prof. Porpiglia comments: "Vascular impressions of the renal collecting system are a common finding on urography. Most are asymptomatic. In 1966 Frayley descibed a rare

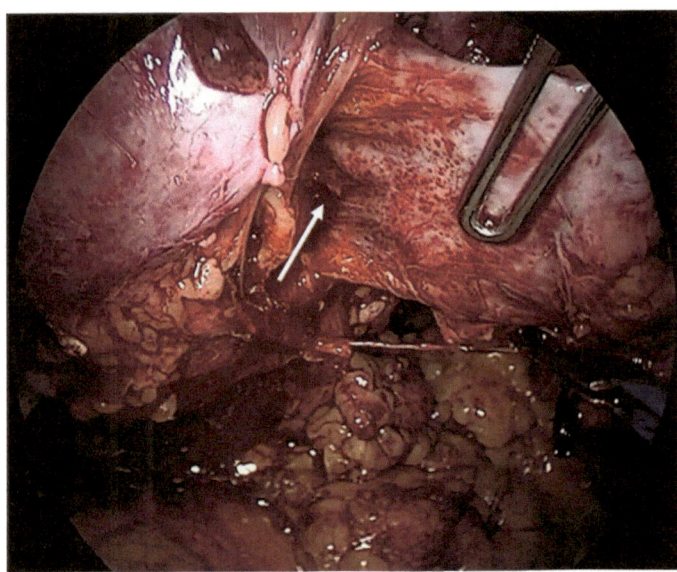

FIGURE 7.43 A vessel crossing at the left upper pole infundibulum resulting in a hydronephrosis: a smooth dissection of the calyx (*white arrow*) is performed without any clamping of segmental branches presenting the thin layer of renal parenchyma of the upper pole of the kidney. Intraoperative laparoscopic photo (courtesy of Prof. F. Porpiglia)

anatomic variant of the renal vasculature that compresses the upper pole infundibulum, resulting in calyceal obstruction and dilation, with symptoms of flank pain and hematuria. If observed via urography, the diagnosis of Fraley's syndrome is confirmed by the finding of a well-defined filling effect in the infundibulum, caused by crossing vessel compression. The upper calyx looks distended. Various treatment methods have been employed successfully to eliminate symptoms, usually requiring surgical exploration. Different open nephron-sparing approaches were described by several authors. To date, descriptions of nephron-sparing laparoscopy or robot-assisted correction techniques of Fraley's syndrome are anecdotal. The nephon-sparing technique is based on the

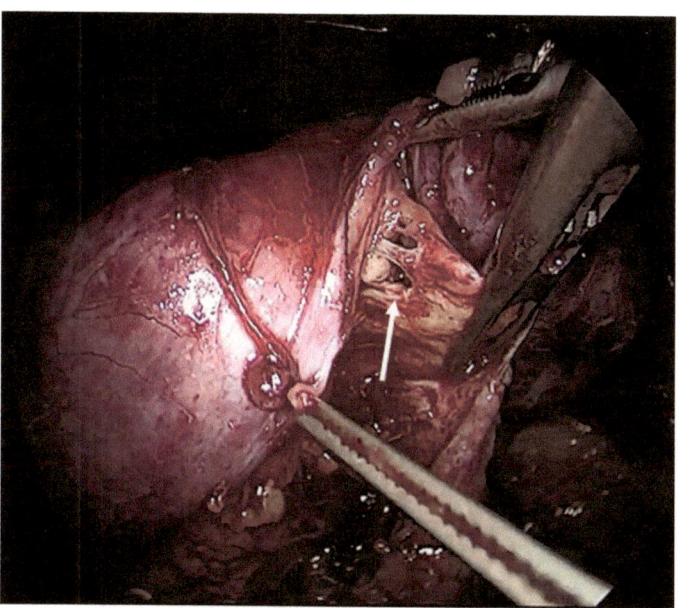

Figure 7.44 A vessel crossing vessel the left upper pole infundibu-lum resulting in a hydronephrosis: in the deepest phase of calycec-tomy the renal papilla and the sinus fat are identified and the smooth muscular fibers of the anchoring calyx are dissected (*white arrow*). Intraoperative laparoscopic photo (courtesy of Prof. F. Porpiglia)

anatomical principle of the segmental distribution of the renal lobes (medullary pyramids and their own calyx). According to this concept it is possible to describe the cali-cectomy, characterized by hilar access, renal sinus explora-tion, and isolation of a specific anatomical segment/lobe. The interlobar vessels are located between different lobes, and should be considered independent from calyceal structures during the surgery, and in fact, if the calicectomy is performed without the clamping of renal branches the parenchymal ischemia is avoided. In the meantime, the preservation of renal tissue surrounding the calyx preserves the intrasinusal segmental artery flow, avoiding their accidental closure by hemostatic sutures."

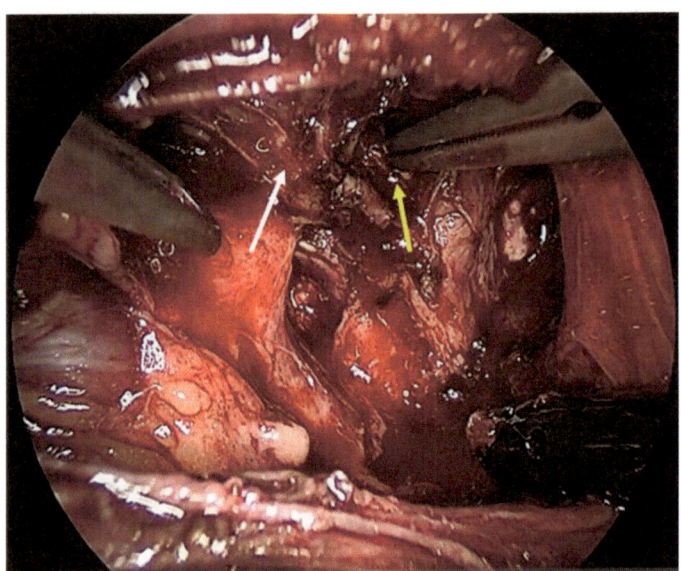

FIGURE 7.45 A vessel crossing *at the left upper* pole infundibulum resulting in a hydronephrosis: at the end of the extirpative phase, the upper pole sinusal cavity is examined in order to identify parenchymal structures like renal papillae and columns of Bertin (*white arrow*). The interlobar vessel is selectively coagulated (*yellow arrow*) avoiding an intrasinusal hematoma. Intraoperative laparoscopic photo (courtesy of Prof. F. Porpiglia)

The sequence of the two cases is very interesting, considering that in the first case the calyx was accomplished through a nephrotomy, i.e., from the outer surface of the kidney, while in the second case there was an endosinusal access for individualization, preparation, and management of the pelvis, calyces, and target vessels. The Frayley syndrome operation was an entirely endorenal surgery, as specified in Chap. 1.

Prof. Porpiglia has these general comments: "In the last 20 years laparoscopy was proposed as a minimally invasive technique in calyceal diverticula. Nowadays robotics has a role in the treatment of this kind of disease too. These minimally invasive approaches, if compared with endourologic

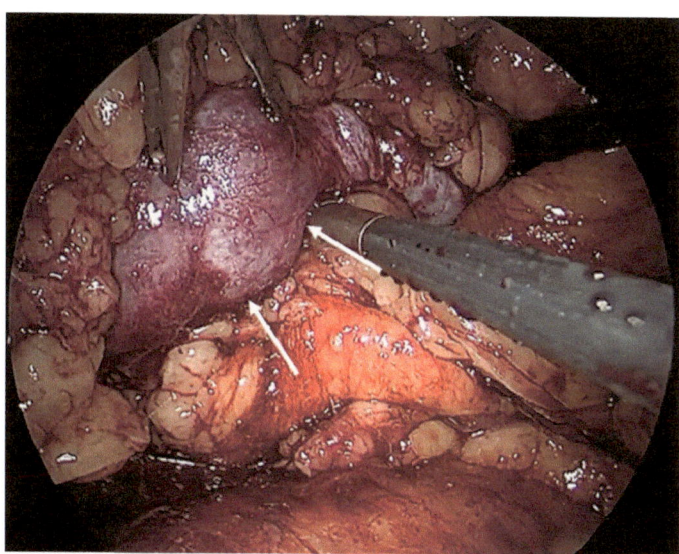

Figure 7.46 A crossing vessel at the left upper pole infundibulum resulting in a hydronephrosis: to complete the procedure the perirenal fat is inserted inside the cavity (*white arrow*) and fixed with PDS 2/0 in order to prevent the risk of bleeding and urinary fistulas. Intraoperative laparoscopic photo (courtesy of Prof. F. Porpiglia)

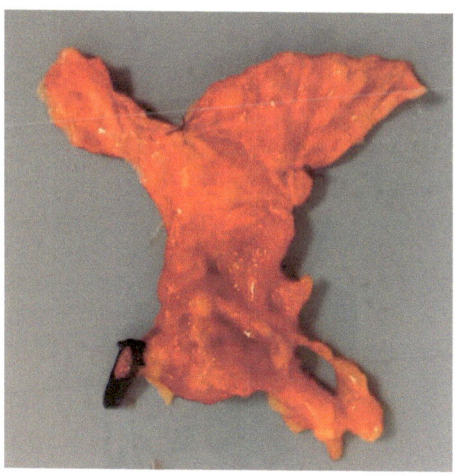

Figure 7.47 A vessel crossing at the left upper pole infundibulum resulting in a hydronephrosis: anatomical specimen of the calycectomy (courtesy of Prof. Porpiglia)

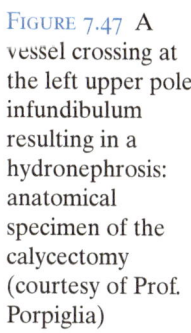

techniques, represent an effective alternative because they allow the treatment of stones and anatomical abnormalities at the same time. They are cavities without significant overlaying renal tissue or without an endoscopically inaccessible infundibulum. Indeed, with these minimally invasive techniques it is possible to obtain a total excision of the diverticulum/hydrocalyx and stones removal, avoiding the risk of recurrence thanks to a complete closure of the diverticular infundibulum."

Notwithstanding these potential advantages, some technical aspects should be kept in mind before embarking on such a procedure. Intraoperative US guidance is essential to define the calyx anatomy and position. Moreover, the renal pedicle should be dissected before starting the nephrotomy in order to identify and manage the renal artery in case of massive bleeding from the parenchyma. Each case has different anatomical details and the surgical strategy must be defined step by step. For this reason, consistent surgical experience in minimally invasive approaches is mandatory.

In this scenario open surgery maintained a marginal role because of its invasiveness. It is still considered when the experience of the surgeon in minimally invasive approaches is limited to date, professor Porpiglia.

Carmelo Boccafoschi, head of the Urology Department of Alessandria Clinic, Alessandria, Italy, very kindly sent me some comments regarding cases of cystic nephroma, pelvic lymphangiomatosis, intrarenal refluxes, and incommon intrarenal operations. He also gave me very interesting intraoperative photographs in open surgery of a special intrarenal access for a minicalico-pyelotomy in order to remove a difficult calyceal stone (Figs. 7.48, 7.49, 7.50, 7.51, 7.52, 7.53, and 7.54). The interest of the case concerns the ability of reaching the calyx and its stone through a minimum nephrotomy at the hilum level. The small opening of the renal sinus was obtained by pulling on the suture threads of the parenchyma cut, which also ensured hemostasis.

Alessandro Volpe, head of the Urological Department and Director of postgraduate School of Urology at East Piedmont

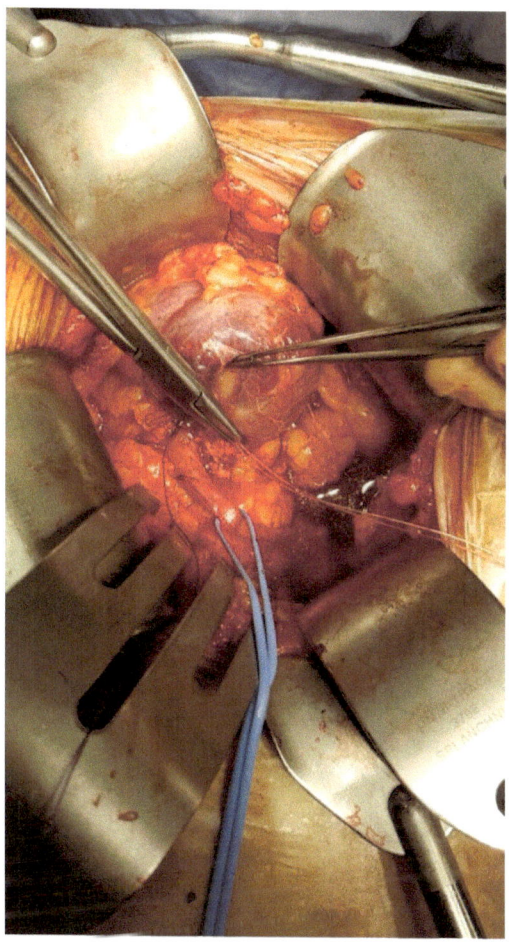

FIGURE 7.48 Open surgery; difficult calyceal stone, showing micro-endorenal pyelo-calicotomy. Intraoperative photo (courtesy of Dr. C. Boccafoschi)

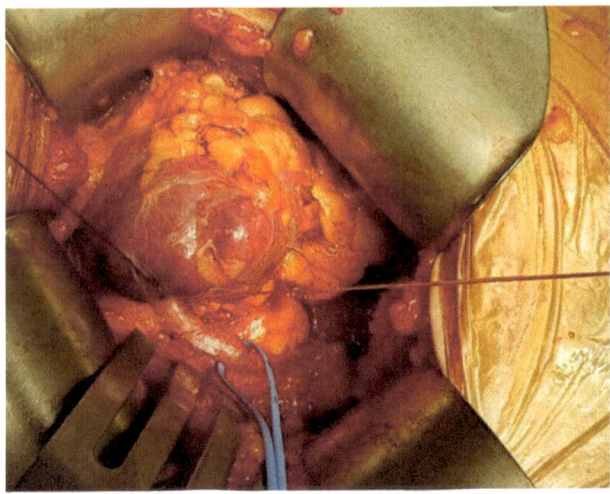

FIGURE 7.49 Open surgery, difficult calyceal stone, showing micro-nephrotomy for sinus access and traction on nephrotomy treads. Intraoperative photo (courtesy of Dr. C. Boccafoschi)

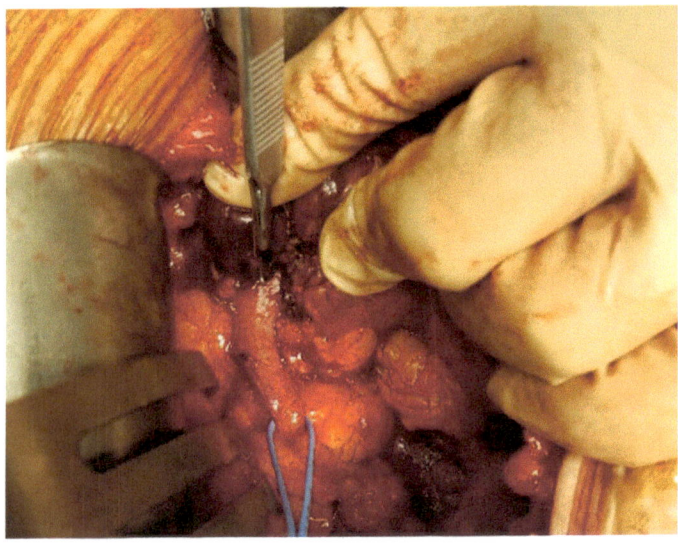

FIGURE 7.50 Open surgery, difficult calyceal stone, showing target calicotomy. Intraoperative photo (courtesy of Dr. C. Boccafoschi)

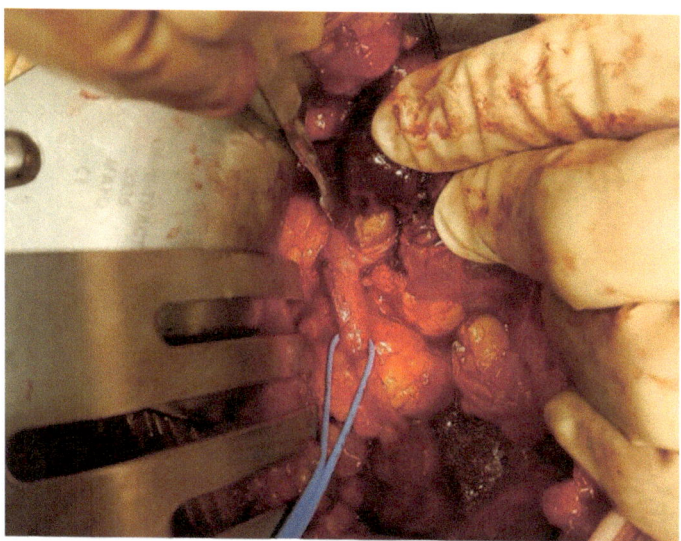

FIGURE 7.51 Open surgery, difficult calyceal stone: stone detachment from the mucosa. Intraoperative photo (courtesy of Dr. C. Boccafoschi)

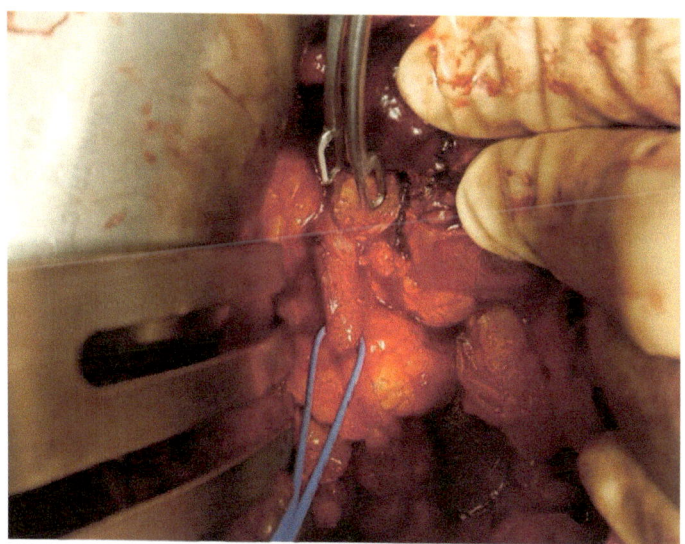

FIGURE 7.52 Open surgery, difficult calyceal stone: stone removing. Intraoperative photo (courtesy of Dr. C. Boccafoschi)

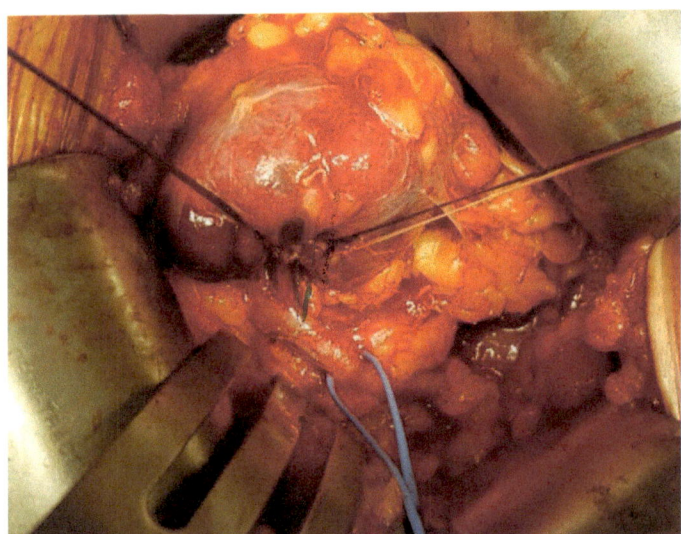

FIGURE 7.53 Open surgery, difficult calyceal stone: pyelo-calyceal cut. Intraoperative photo (courtesy of Dr. C. Boccafoschi)

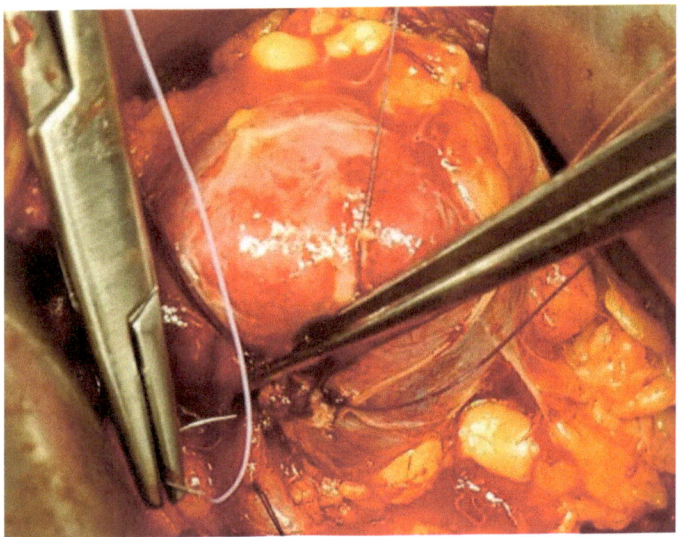

FIGURE 7.54 Open surgery, difficult calyceal stone: suture of the pyelo-calycotomy. Intraoperative photo (courtesy of Dr. C. Boccafoschi)

University, Novara, Italy, assured me that partial nephrectomies can be executed robotically and kindly sent me many
intraoperative photographs of a robotic-assisted partial
nephrectomy for a localized tumor of the kidney, in order to
demonstrate details of all the special techniques, starting from
the patient position, portae topography, renal parenchyma cutting, exploring, suturing, and so on (Figs. 7.53, 7.54, 7.55, 7.56,
7.57, and 7.58). Prof. Volpe has no doubts that renal segmentectomy can also be executed robotically (Figs. 7.59 and 7.60).

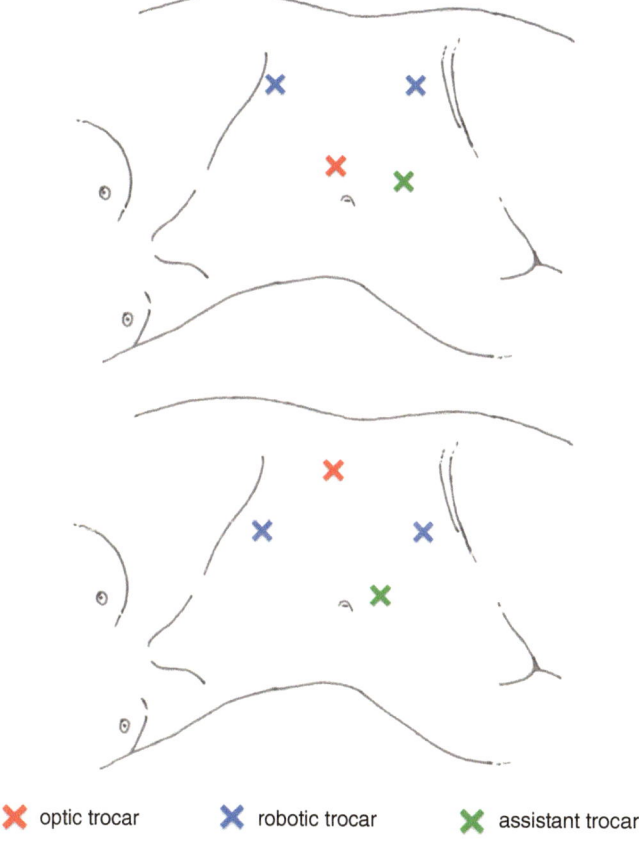

❌ optic trocar   ❌ robotic trocar   ❌ assistant trocar

FIGURE 7.55 Robotic surgery: medial (**a**) and lateral (**b**) camera trocar placement (courtesy of Prof. A. Volpe)

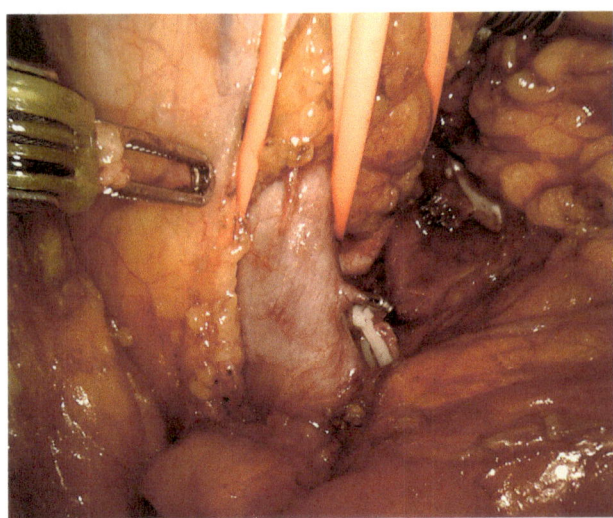

FIGURE 7.56 Robotic surgery: hilar control. A vessel loop is passed around the renal vein and secured with a Hem-o-lok clip. Intraoperative photo (courtesy of Prof. A. Volpe)

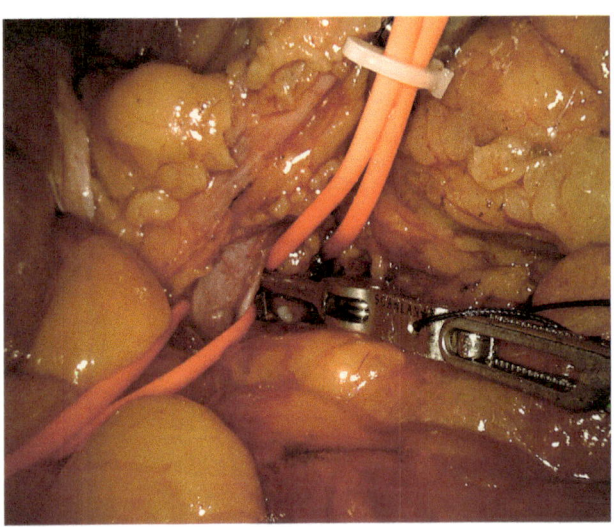

FIGURE 7.57 Robotic surgery: clamping of the renal artery with a robotic bulldog clip. Intraoperative photo (courtesy of Prof. A. Volpe)

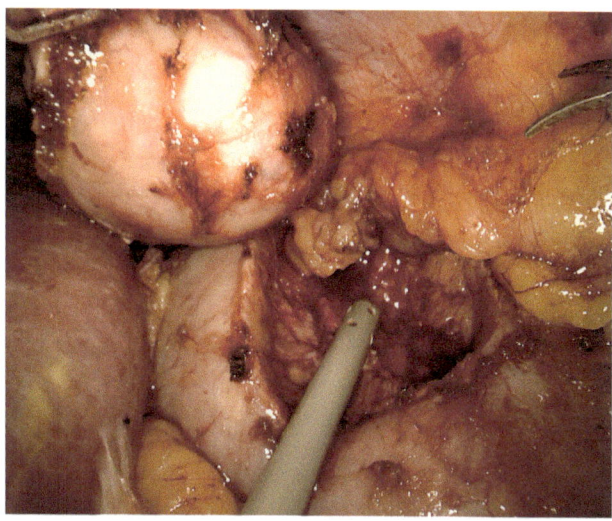

FIGURE 7.58 Robotic surgery: tumor excision using monopolar curved scissors (see Fig. 1.6) and residual parenchymal inspection. Intraoperative photo (courtesy of Prof. A. Volpe)

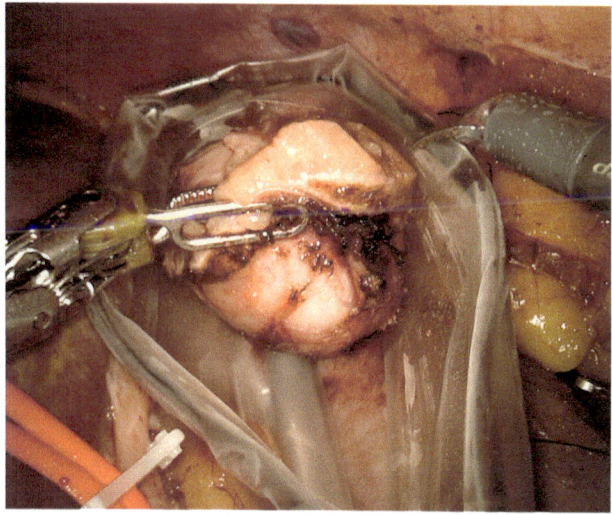

FIGURE 7.59 Robotic surgery: placement of the excised renal tumor in an endobag. Intraoperative photo (courtesy of Prof. A. Volpe)

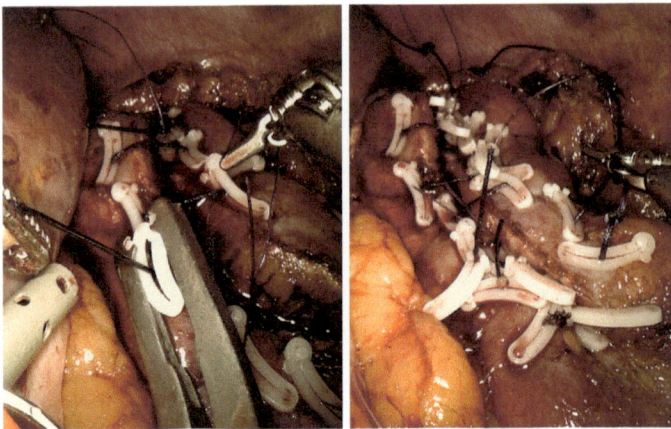

FIGURE 7.60 Outer renography performed using a polifilament 1–0 suture, using a sliding clip technique. Intraoperative photo (courtesy of Prof. A. Volpe)

References

1. Zizmv AR, Evan AP, Coe FL, Worcester EM. Do kidney stone formers have a kidney disease? Kidney Int. 2015;88:1240–9.
2. Evan AP, Coe FL, Lingeman JE, et al. Mehanism of formation of human calcium oxalate stones on randall's plaque. Anat Rec (Hoboken). 2007;290:1315–23.
3. Evan AP, Lingeman JE, Coe FL, et al. Role of interatitial apatite plaque in the pathogenesis of the common calcium oxalate stone. Semin Nephrol. 2008;28:111–9.
4. Ingram CJE, Muller Yvalitan CA, Swallw MGT. Lactose digestion and evolutionary genetics of lactose persistence. Hum Genet. 2009;124:579–91.
5. Rocca Rossetti S. La Terapia della Calcolosi Urinaria. Conferenza VI Congresso Nazionale CLU, Srt, Torino: In; 2015.
6. Vent A, Guner MD. Helicobacter pylory and urinary system stones. Endoluminal damage as subhypothesis to support the current stone theory. Med Hypotheses. 2014;83(6):677–80.
7. Stoller MI, Meng MI, Abramahams MH, Kane JP. The primary stone event: a new vascular etiology. J Urol. 2004;171:1920–4.
8. Smith GM, Zwart SR, et al. Men and women in the space: bone loss and kidney risk after long duration spaceflight. J Bone Miner Res. 2024;29(6):1639–45.
9. Liskopoulos V. The kidney in the space. In: 6th international conference of aerospace medicine, Thessaloniki, Set; 2010.
10. Deng E, et al. Study of histopathological and molecular changes of rat kidney under simulated weightlessness and resistance training protective effect. PLoS One. 2011;6(5):e20008.
11. Blaser MJ, Falow WS. What are the consequenses of the disappering human microbiota? Nat Rev Microbiol. 2009;7(12):857–94.

12. Moe OO. Kidney stones: phatophysiology and medical menagement. Lancet. 2006;367:333–44.
13. Khan SR, Canales BR. Unified theory on the pathogenesis of randall plaques and plugs. Urolithiasis. 2015;41(Suppl 11):109–23.
14. Staelher W. Recent changes in the assesment in urogenital tuberculosis. Int Urol Nephrol. 1975;7(4):277–88.
15. Takahashi S, Takeyama K, et al. Current survey of urinary tuberculosis in Kokkaido, Japan. J Infect Chemother. 2007;13:105–8.
16. Singh DD, Vogel M, Muller-Stover I, et al. Tb or not Tb? Difficulties in the diagnostic of tuberculosis in HIV-negative immigranrs in Germany. Eur J Med Res. 2011;16(9):381.
17. European Center for Disease Prevention and Control. Tuberculosis surbeillance and monitoring in Europe; 2016.
18. Ministero della Salute. La Tubercolosi in Italia. Rapporto; 2008.
19. Istituto Superiore di Sanità. Istituto Nazionale di Statistica. La mortalità in Italia nell'anno 2001. p. 16.
20. Merchant S, Bahharati A, Merchant N. Tuberculosis of the genito-urinary system-urinary tract tuberculosis: renal tuberculosis, part. I. Indian J Radiol Imaging. 2013;23(1):46–63.
21. Semb C. The selective principle in the treatment of renal tucerculosis. J Oslo City Hosp. 1953;3:45.
22. Semb C. Conservative renal surgery. J Roy Coll Surg Edinb. 1964;10:9–30.
23. Gow G. Partial nephrectomy. Lancet. 1959;274:759–61.
24. Gow G. Genito-urinary tuberculosis: a study of 700 cases. Lancet. 1963;282:261–5.
25. Gow G. Renal calcifications in genito-urinary tuberculosis. Br J Surg. 1965;52(4):283–8.
26. Gow G. Results of treatment in a large series of renal tuberculosis. Br J Urol. 1970;48:4–15.
27. Gow G. Genito urinary tuberculosis. In: Blandy J, editor. Urology, vol. I, Chap. 12. Edinburg: Blackwell Scientific Publications; 1985. p. 226 e sgg.
28. Siegel A. Anatomic basis of partial nephrectomy. Urol Int. 1964;11:15–74.
29. Henley HG. Conservative surgery in renal tuberculosis. Br J Urol. 1961;48:415–20.
30. Krishnamoopthy S, Gopolascrisham G. Surgical management of renal tuberculosis. Indian J Urol. 2008;24(3):369.
31. Cek M, Lenk S, and al. Guidlines for Management of Genito-Urinary Tuberculosis. Eur Urol. 2005;49(3): 353–62
32. Cupta NP, Kumar R, Mumadada OP, Aron M, Kemal AK, Dogra PN, Seth A. Reconstructive surgery for the management of

genito-urinaty tuberculosis: a single center experience. J Urol. 2006;175(6):2150–4.

33. Editorial Comment, idem, p. 2154.

34. Carl P, Stark L. Indication for surgical management of genito-urinary tuberculosis. World J Surg. 1997;21(5):505–10.

35. Henley HG. Cavernotomy and partial nephrectomy in renal tuberculosis. Br J Urol. 1970;46(6):661–6.

36. Crow JC, Cosbie Ross J, Still Hill CA. Partial nephrectomy: a critical study. Lancet. 1959;274(7106):59–61.

37. Cerulli N, De Angelis S, Sebastiani A. Genito-urinary tuberculosis. In: Cerulli N, De Angeli S, Sebastiani A, editors. Tropical renal and urological diseases. Milano: Wichting Publisher; 1996. p. 50 and sgg.

38. Verswiivel G, Jansen F, Vandenvenne J, Stenssens L, Mavlaerts P, Palmers Y. Renal macronodular tuberculoma. CT and MR findings in an asyntomatic patient. J Belg Radiol. 2002;85(4):203–5.

39. Murata Y, Yamada I, Sumya Y, Schichio Y, Suzuki Y. Abdominal macronodular tuberculoma: MR findings. J Comput Assest Tomogr. 1996;20(4):643–6.

40. Soica S, Damian A, Otean I, Malica G. Results obtained with the dug and surgical treatment of exclusive renal tuberculoma with uni or bilateral polar localization. Rev Med Chir Soc Med Nat Iasi. 1985;1:57–9.

41. Chen RY, Chan H. Renal dysplasia. Arch Pathol Lab Med. 2015;139(4):547–50.

42. Bernstein J, Arant BS Jr, Garel L, Stickler GB, Neal IV, Bagenstoss AH. Renal dysplasia and cystic diseases. Pediatr Nephrol. 1992:357–67.

43. Centi S. Identificazione di Patterns di Espressione Genica della Displasia Renale Associata ad Uropatia Malformativa. Scuola di Dottorato di Ricerca di Medicina dello Sviluppo e Scienza di Programmazione dell'Università di Padova. 2008;31:01.

44. Bezzi E. Urologia. Malformazioni Renali. Torino: UTET; 1974. p. 137–238.

45. Taka S, Yamagiki I, et al. The incidence of simple renal cyst by computed tomography. Clin Radiol. 1983;34(4):437–9.

46. Rankin EB, Tomasgewoki JE, Haase VH. Renal cyst development in mice with conditional inactivation of the von Hiooel-Lindau tumor suppressor. Cancer Res. 2006;66:2576–83.

47. Joshi VV, Freepath MD, Brace Beewith J. Multilobular cyst of the kidney (cystic nephroma), and cystic, partially differntiated nephroblastoma. Terminology and criteria for diagnosis. Cancer. 1989;64:466–79.

48. Dunnil MS, Millard PR, Oliver D. Acquired cystic disease of the kidneys: a hazard of long-term intermittent maintenance haemodialysis. J Clin Pathol. 1977;30:868–77.

49. Murad T, Komaiko W, Oyan R, Bauer K. Multilocular cystic renal cell carcinoma. Am J Clin Pathol. 1991;95(5):633–7.

50. Bosniak MA. The current radiologic approach to renal cysts. Radiology. 1986;158:1–10.

51. Amar AD, Das S. Surgical management of benign renal cysts causing obstruction of renal pelvis. Urology. 1984;24(5):429–33.

52. Sampson JR, Maheeshwar MM, et al. Renal cystic disease in tuberous sclerosis: role of the polycystic kidney disease 1 gene. Am J Hum Genet. 1977;61:843–51.

53. Corica FA, Iczkowski KA, et al. Cystic renal cell carcinoma is cured by resection: a study of 24 cases with long-term followup. J Urol. 1999;161(2):408–11.

54. Suzigan S, Lopez-Beltrain A, et al. Multilocular cystic renal cell carcinoma: a report of 45 cases of a kidney tumor of low malignant potential. Am J Clin Pathol. 2006;125(2):217–22.

55. Silverman SG, Koseraud K, et al. Hyperattenuating renal masses: etiologies, pathogenesis and imaging evaluation. Radiographics. 2007;27(4):1131–43.

56. Laucis SP, Melachan MSF. Aging and simple cyst of the kidney. Br J Radiol. 2014;54(637):12–4.

57. Marques DT, Bezena RO, et al. Spontaneous combined rupture of a pelvicalyceal cyst into the collector system and retroperitoneal space during the acquisition of the computed tomography scan images: a case report. J Case Rep. 2012;6(1):386.

58. Baert L, Steg A. On the pathogenesis of simple renal cysts in the adult. A microdissection Study. Urol Res. 1977;5(3):103–8.

59. A. Presenti Gritti, A. Bolletta. Le Malattie del Ciglio. Rene Policistico. G.I.N. (Giorn. Ital. Nefrol.) Ott; 2015. 34,1.

60. Hikdembrandt F, Attanasio M, Otto E. Nephronophthisis disease mechanisms of a ciliopathy. JASN. 2009;30(1):23–5.

61. Sung L, Miller JJ, et al. Mapping the NPHP-JBTS-MKS protein network renal ciliopathy disease gene and pathways. Cell. 2011;145(4):513–29.

62. Leva G, Annoscia S, Lozzi C, Montefiore F, Di Mauro A, Graci E, Boccafoschi C. Nefroma cistico: nostra esperienza su due casi e revisione della letteratura. Arch Ital Urol. 1990;LVII:317–22.

63. Marino G, Surleti D, Laudi M, Motta M, Mosso L, Ravarino M, Torchio B. Nefroma cistico multiloculare del rene. Descrizione

di un caso e considerazioni cliniche. Rivista Internazionale di Cultura Urologica. 2008;75(2):5–10.

64. Cevoli R, Torchio B, Buffa G, Tartagkio S, Pacilio N. Benign multilocular cystic nephroma. Description of 1 case. Minerva urologica e nefrologica. 1998;41(2):127–30.

65. Boccafoschi C. Comunicazione Personale (in press).

66. Suzigan S, Lopez-Beltrain A, et al. Multilocular cystic renal cell carcinoma: a report of 45 cases of a kidney tumor of low malignant potential. Am J Clin Pathol. 2006;125(2):217–22.

67. Corica FA, Iczkowski KA, et al. Cystic renal cell carcinoma is cured by resection: a study of 24 cases with long-term followup. J Urol. 1999;161(2):408–11.

68. Murad T, Komaiko W, Oyan R, Bauer K. Multilocular cystic renal cell carcinoma. Am J Clin Pathol. 1991;95(5):633–7.

69. Joshi VV, Freepath MD, Brace Beewith J. Multilobular cyst of the kidney (cystic nephroma), and cystic, partially differentiated nephroblastoma. Terminology and criteria for diagnosis. Cancer. 1989;64:466–15.

70. Rocca Rossetti S. I Tumori Urologici. In: Veronesi U, editor. Trattato di Oncologia Chirurgica, vol. II. UTET; 1989. p. 625.

71. Powell T, Schackman R, Johnson HD. Multilocular cysts of the kidney: report of five case with review of the literature. J Clin Pathol. 1976;65:93.

72. Punia RPS, Mohan H, Bal A, Komar Bansal W. Unilateral and segmental cystic disease of the kidney. Int J Urol. 2006;12:308–10.

73. Wel Lara B, Ibanez Martinez J, Garzia Gonzalez I, Bedova Belmonte JJ. Unilateral neonatal cystic disease of the kidney as first manifestation of tuberous sclerosis. Arch Esp Urol. 1997;50(9):1012–4.

74. Molino D, Sepe J, A Anastasio P, De Santo N. The history of von Hippel Lindau discase. J Nephrol. 2006;19(Suppl 10):S119–23.

75. Menko FH, Manher EK. Diagnosis and management of hereditary renal cell cancer. Recent Results Cancer Res. 2016;205:85–104.

76. Kerr LA, Blute ML, Ryu H, Swensten SJ, Malek RS. Renal angiomyolipoma in association with pulmonary lymphangioleimyomatosis, forme fruste of tuberous sclerosis. Urology. 1993;41(5):440–4.

77. Chattergee J, Heinder W, Vorreuther R, Engelman U, Lackner R. Recurrent bleeding of angiomyolipomas in tuberous sclerosis. Urol Int. 1996;56(1):44–7.

78. Mettin RR, Hirsch A, Kless W, Sirbe S. Wide spectrum of clinical manifestations in children with tuberous sclerosis complex. Follow up of 20 children. Brain Dev. 2014;36(4):306–14.
79. Sampson JR, Maheeshwar MM, et al. Renal cystic disease in tuberous sclerosis: Role of the polycystic kidney disease 1 gene. Am J Hum Genet. 1977;61:843–51.
80. Hansinghani MG, Manher MM, et al. Incidence of malignancy in complex cystic renal masses (Bosniak category (III)): should imaging-guided biopsy precede surgery. Am J Roentgenol. 2003;180(3):755–8.
81. Silverman SG, Koseraud K, et al. Hyperattenuating renal masses: etiologies, pathogenesis and imaging evaluation. Radiographics. 2007;27(4):1131–43.
82. Well LB, Ibanez MJ, Garcia GI, Bedoya BJ. Unilateral neonatal cystic disease of the kidney as first manifestation of tuberous sclerosis. Arch Esp Urol. 1997;50(9):1012–4.
83. Suzuki K, Kurokawa S, Muraiski O, et al. Segmental multicystic dysplastic kidney in adult men. Urol Int. 2001;66:51–4.
84. Kalyoussel E, Hwang J, Frasad V, Barone J. Segmental multicystic dysplastic kidney in children. Urology. 2016;68(5):1121–9.
85. Han JH, Lee YS, Kim MJ, Lee MJ, Im YJ, Hau SW. Conservative management of segmental multicystic dysplastic kidney in children. Urology. 2015;86(5):1013–8.
86. Cardona Grau D, Cogan BA. Update on multicystic dysplastic kidney. Curr Urol Rep. 2015;16(10):67.
87. Caliaway AC, Whittam B, et al. Multicystic dysplastic kidney: is an initial voiding cystourethrogram necessary? Can J Urol. 2014;21(5):7510–4.
88. Bernstein J, Arant AS, et al. Renal dysplasia and cystic disease. Pediatr Nephrol. 1984; 533–67. (Proceeding of 6th international Symposium of Pediatric Nephrology. Hannover 29th August–2nd September, 1984).
89. Çopez JJ, Larrinage G, Angulo JC. The normal and pathologic renal medulla: a comprehensive overview. Pathol Res Pract. 2015;211(4):271–80.
90. R. Cacchi, V. Ricci. Su una rara e forse non ancora descritta affezione cistica delle piramidi renali: rene a spugna. Atti SIU, 1049, 21, 59.
91. Cacchi R, Ricci V. Sur une maladie kistique multiple des pyramides renales: "Le Rein en Spogne". J Urol Néphrol. 1949;55:49.

92. Lenarduzzi G. La forma circoscritta del rene a spugna. Radiol Med. 1951;37:776.
93. Pansadoro V. Su un caso di malattia cistica multipla delle piramidi, renali o rene a spugna. Quaderni di Urol. 1952;1:124–38.
94. Palubinskas AJ. Medullary sponge kidney. Radiology. 1961;76(6):911–9.
95. Petter EL, Osathanondh V. Medullary sponge kidney. Two cases in young infants. J Pediatr. 1963;62:901–7.
96. Curtis Morris R, Yamauchi H, Palubinskas AJ, Honwenstine H. Medullary sponge kidney. Am J Med. 1965;38(6):883–92.
97. Di Egidio F, et al. Imaging nel rene a spugna midollare: nota per l'urologo. Urologia. 2014;81(4):196–9.
98. Fabris A, Bruschi M, et al. Proteomic-based research strategy identified laminin subunit alpha 2 as potential urinary-specific biomarker for medullary sponge kidney disease. Kidney. 2017;91(2):459–68.
99. Slaats GG, Lilian MR, Giles RH. Nephonophthisis: should we target cyst or fibrosis. Pediatr Nephrol. 2016;31(14):545–54.
100. Kuraishi FM, Ngo TT, Iolael GM, Dahal NK. CT urography for diagnosis of medullary sponge kidney. Am J Nephrol. 2014;39(2):165–76.
101. Hida T, Nischie A, et al. MR imaging of focal medullary sponge kidney: case report. Magn Reson Med Sci. 2012;11(1):65–9.
102. Pianezza ML, Estey EP. Laparoscopic removal of a pelvic cyst associated with obstructed megaureter and dysplastic renal remnant. Can Urol Assoc. 2009;3(2):159–62.
103. Marques DT, Bezena RO, et al. Spontaneous combined rupture of a pelvicalyceal cyst into the collecting system and retroperitoneal space during the acquisition of the computed tomography scan images: a case report. J Med Case Rep. 2012;6(1):366.
104. Arant BS Jr, Sotelo-Avila C, Bernstein J. Segmental "Hypoplasia" ows microcysts and glomerular absence or paucity; the ask-upmark kidney. J Pediatr. 1079;93:931–8.
105. Shindo S, Bernstein J, Arant RS. Evolution of segmental atrophy (ask-upmark kidney) in children with vesicoureteric reflux: radiographic and morphologic study. J Pediatr. 1984;102(6):847–54.
106. Lyungqwist A, Lagergren C. The ask-upmark kideny. A congenital renal anomaly studied by micro-angiography and histology. Acta Pathol Microbiol Scand. 1962;56(3):277–83.

107. Rosenfeld JB, Cohen L, Garty J, Ben Bassat M. Unilateral renal hypoplasia with hypertension (ask-upmark kidney). Br Med J. 1973;2:217–8.

108. Babin J, Sacjett M, Delange C, Label M. The ask-upmark kidney: a curable cause of hypertension in young patients. J Hum Hypertens. 2005;19(4):315–6.

109. Amaur A, Adami J, Abbar M. Segmental renal hypoplasia or ask-upmark kidney. Anatomopathologic approach: report of 2 cases. Ann Urol. 2003;37(1):1–4.

110. Lenley KV, Kriz W. Anatomy of the renal interstitium- symposoim on the cell biology of the tubulum interstitium. Kidney Int. 1991;38:370–81.

111. Aleckovic-Allovic A, Nel D, Wovwod A. Granulomatous interstitial nephritis: a chameleon in a globalized world. Clin Kidney J. 2015;8(5):611–5.

112. Shah S, Carter-Monroe N, Atta MG. Granulomatous interstitial nephritis. Clin Kidney J. 2015;8(5):516–23.

113. Agraval V, Kaul A, Prassad N, Sharma K, Agarwal W. Etiological diagnosis of granulomatous tubulointerstitial nephritis in tropics. Clin Kidney J. 2015;8(5):524–30.

114. Basel MA, Nebeeh A, Atwan N. Granulomatous pyelonephritis in bilhartial patients: a report of 25 cases. J Urol. 1989;141:261.

115. Ballestreros SJ. Inusuales formas clinicas de presentacion y associaciones patològicas raras de pielonefritis granulomatosa. Arch Esp Urol. 2002;55(2):119–90.

116. Busta Castaron L, Gòmez Castro A, Candell Alononso J, Gonsalez Martin M. Xantogranulomatous pyelonephritis (and cystic dysplasia) in a newborn. Arch Esp Urol. 1980;33(2):303–14.

117. Cerulli N, De Angelis S, Sebastiani A. Tropical renal and urological diseases. Milano: Whichtig; 1996. p. 124–42.

118. Puigvert A. Disembriogenia de l'estrem terminal del conduct de kupfer. Comunicaciò presentada el die 18 de Febrier de 1965.

119. Rigaud J, Catelinau X, Vasse N, Karan G, Buzelin JM, Buchet O. Lumbar pain and hydrocalyx. Progres en urologie: journal de l'Association francaise d'urologie et de la Societe francaise d'urologie. 2011;11(3):498–501.

120. Frong D, Gotz F, Hubler J, Nagy Z. Surgery of calculus hydrocalyx (calicoplastic surgery). Int Urol Nephrol. 1987;19(2):129–35.

121. Anastasov G, Petkov A. Hydrocalyx (Fraley's Syndrome). Vŭtreshni bolesti. 1977;16(3):89–93.
122. Stuart Wolf J Jr. Caliceal diverticulum and hydrocalyx: laparoscopic management. Urol Clin North Am. 2000;77(4):655–60.
123. Dorsey JW. Solitary hydrocalyx secondary to a dumbbell calculus. J Urol. 1949;62(5):743–7.
124. Ataka JH, Pikindil G, Alagol B, Inci O. A new cause of curvilinear renal calcification: calcified hydrocalycosis. Eur J Radiol. 2000;35(1):16–9.
125. Timmons JW Jr, Maleck RS, Hattery RR, Deweerd JH. Caliceal diverticulum. J Urol. 1975;114(2):6–9.
126. Karzmazin B, Kaifer M, Jernings SG, Mumala R, Raske ME. Caliceal diverticulum in pediatric patients: the spectrum of imaging findings. Pediatr Radiol. 2011;41(11):1369–73.
127. Rapp DE, Gerber GS. Management of caliceal diverticula. J Endourol. 2004;18(9):805–10.
128. Monga M, Smith R, Ferral H, Thomas R. Percutaneous ablation of caliceal diverticulum: Long term followup. J Urol. 1995;153(6):1878–81.
129. Grasso M, Lamg G, Loesidws P, Bagley D, Taylor F. Endoscopic management of the symptomatic caliceal diverticular calculus. J Urol. 1995;153(6):1878–81.
130. Ruckle HC, Segura JW. Laparoscopic treatment of a stone filled caliceal diverticulum: a definitive, minimally invasive therapeutic option. J Urol. 1994;15(1):122–4.
131. Basiri A, Radfar MH, Lashay A. Laparoscopic management of caliceal diverticulum: our experience, literature review and pooling analysis. J Endourol. 2013;27(5):283–6.
132. Timmons JW Jr, Maleck RS, Hattery RR, Deweerd JH. Caliceal diverticulum. J Urol. 1975;114(2):6–9.
133. Karzmazin B, Kaifer M, Jernings SG, Mumala R, Raske ME. Caliceal diverticulum in pediatric patients: the spectrum of imaging findings. Pediatr Radiol. 2011;41(11):1369–73.
134. Rapp DE, Gerber GS. Management of caliceal diverticula. J Endourol. 2004;18(9):805–10.
135. Monga M, Smith R, Ferral H, Thomas R. Percutaneous ablation of caliceal diverticulum: long term followup. J Urol. 1995;153(6):1878–81.
136. Grasso M, Lamg G, Loesidws P, Bagley D, Taylor F. Endoscopic management of the symptomatic caliceal diverticular calculus. J Urol. 1995;153(6):1878–81.

137. Ruckle HC, Segura JW. Laparoscopic treatment of a stone filled caliceal diverticulum: a definitive, minimally invasive therapeutic option. J Urol. 1994;15(1):122–4.

138. Picardi N, Fidotti E. Megapolycalicosis in the picture of kidney pelvis diseases. Diagnosis and therapeutic problems. Ann Ital Chir. 1971;41(1):3–20.

139. Castelli S, Domenici R, Galli S. Megapolycalicosis. Report of a new case. Minerva Pediatr. 1983;35(6):291–3.

140. Marsili E, Camerani M, et al. Mega-poly-calicosis. Apropos of a case with prenatal and postnatal diagnosis. J Urol. 1991;97(6):224–37.

141. Galimetzer J, Omobono E. Megapolycalicosis: a case report. Minerva Pediatr. 1994;48(5):221–4.

142. Lee KM, Kim RJ, Lee D-Y. A case of congenital megacalyces. Korean J Pediatr. 1997;40(8):883–6.

143. Bekele W, Sanchez TR. Congenital megacalycosis presenting as neonatal hydronephrosis. Pediatr Radiol. 2010;40(9):1579.

144. Zerin JM. Congenital megacalyces. Pediatr Radiol. 2010;40(9):1470.

145. Boix OR, Buisan RO, et al. Horse shoe kidney with congenital megacalyces and renal stones. Actas Urol Esp. 2006;30(7):731.

146. Boyce WH, Whitehurst AW. Hypoplasia of the major renal conduits. J Urol. 1976;116:352–5.

147. Fraley EE. Vascular obstruction of superior infundibulum causing nephralgia: new syndrome. N Engl J Med. 1966;275:1403–9.

148. Johnston JH, Sandomiski SR. Intrarenal vascular obstruction of the superior infundibulum in children. J Pediatr. 1972;7:318–23.

149. Kabalis PP, Malek RS. Infundibulopelvic stenosis. J Urol. 1981;125(4):568.

150. Hasmnn DA, Kommer SA, Malek RS, Allen TD. Infundibulopelvic stenosis. A long-term followup. J Urol. 1994;152:837–40.

151. Bauer SB. Disginesia infundibulo-pelvica in anomalie del rene e della giunzione pielouretereale. Chap. 58 pp. 1755–56, vol. 4. Walsh, Retic, Vaugham e Wein, Urologia di Campbell, Verducci Ed.; 1999.

152. Craver R, Boyd R, Ward K, Harmon E. Renal hypertrophic infundibular stenosis. Fetal Pediatr Pathol. 2004;23(4):285–92.

153. Tanagho EA. Embriologic basis for lower ureteral anomalies a hypothesis. Urology. 1976;7:451–64.

154. Ohman EL, Borofski MS, Han JS, Huang WC, Shah O. Unusual presentation of ectopic insertion of duplicated collecting system in an adult male. Urology. 2013;8(1):36–7.
155. Bezzi E. Urologia, Malformazioni Renali. Torino: UTET; 1974. p. 177–85.
156. Johnston J. Ureter duplication, Chap. 21, Part 3, p. 543. In: Blandy J, editor. Urology, vol. I. Oxford: Blackwell Scientific Publications; 1976.
157. Boccafoschi C, Lugnani F. Intrarenal reflux. Urol Res. 1995;13:253–8.
158. Carris CK, Dvkhulgen RE. Yo-Yo renal pelvis: an unusual cause of flank pain. J Urol. 1997;117(2):153–5.
159. Shama SK, Susuchi CL, Kumar S, Bagna BC, Suri S. Ureteric diverticula: ureteric-diverticular reflux and Yo-Yo effect. A television study with spot filming. Br J Urol. 1998;52(5):545–7.
160. Tuney D, Akpinar IN, Biren T, Arbal ME, Gurmen N. Inverted Y ureteral anomaly and associated distal Yo-Yo phenomenon. Australas Radiol. 1998;42(2):154–6.
161. Chan KW, Metewel C. Scintigraphic detection of Yo-Yo phenomenon in incomplete ureteric duplication. Pedaitr Radiol. 2003;33(1):59–61.
162. Enoglu M, Unsal A, Cimentape E, Bakirtas H. Giant ureteral stone associated with partial ureteral duplication. Int Urol Nephrol. 2003;35(4):485–7.
163. Pellegrin J. L'Appareil Urinaire dans la Serie Animale. Anatomie, Embriologie e Phisiologie. In: Posson A, Desnos E, editors. Enciclppedie Francaise d'Urologie, vol. tome premier, deuxième partie. Paris: Octave Doin e Fils Ed; 1904. p. 295–364.
164. Williams MF. Morphological evidence of marine adaptation in human kidneys. Med Hypotheses. 2006;66(2):247–57.
165. Rocca Rossetti S. Il Rene Parla: l'Uomo viene dal Mare. Urologia. 2007;74(2):5–7., S1–5.
166. Upadhyay KK, Silverstein DM. Renal development: a complex process dependent on inductive interation. Curr Pediatr Rev. 2014;10(2):107–14.
167. Chan D. The role of pax 2 in regulation of kidney development and disease. Yi Chuan. 2011;33(9):931–8.
168. Kevin VL, Kritz W. Symposium on cell biology of the tubulo interstisium. Anatomy of renal interstitium. Kidney Int. 1991;39:370–81.
169. Puigvert A. Calical urodynamics. Urol Int. 1975;30:282–96.

170. Arias LF, Ortis-Arango N. Intrarenal smooth muscle: histology of a complex urodynamic machine. Axtas Urolog Espan. 2013;37(3):129–34.

171. Lopez JI, Larrinagag G, Kurodan N, Angulo JC. The normal and pathologic renal medulla: a comprehensive overview. Pathology. 2015;211:271–80.

172. Mezzabotta F. The kidney development, repair and regeneration. Kidstem international conference, Liverpool, 17–19 September 2008. G Ital Nefrol. 2009;26(3):297.

173. Graves FT. The vascular anatomy and the principles of intrarenal access. In: Wickham JAE, editor. Intrarenal surgery. London: Churchill-Livingstone; 1984. p. 1–29.

174. Boyce WH. Anatrophic nephrotomy. In: Wickham JAE, editor. Intrarenal surgery; 1984. p. 154–65.

175. Swinney J, Hammerskey DP. Handbook of operative urological surgery. Edinburgh, London: E.C. Livingstone Ltd; 1963. p. 34–5.

176. Rocca Rossetti S. Le calicectomie. Trieste: Relazione SUNI; 1976.

177. Rocca Rossetti S. Intrarenal plastic surgery for the collecting system. In: Proceedings international symposium. Wien: Ed. Porpacsy 133; 1979.

178. Rocca Rossetti S. Malformazioni urinarie. In: Trattato di tecnica chirurgica. Chirurgia Urologica. Torino: UTET; 1981. p. 106–134.

179. Costantini A, Turini D. Calicectomie in Chirurgia dei calici e dei peduncoli caliciali. In: Trattato di tecnica chirugica. chirurgia urologica. Torino: UTET; 1981. p. 146.

180. Henle citato da Gil-Vernet [10].

181. Fey B. L'Abord du Rein par la Vie Toracoabdominale. Arch. De la Clinique Necker, 1925;5.

182. Gil-Vernet JM. La cirurgia intrasinusal de los calcolos coralliformes. In: Proceedings of the XVth intern congress of the urological society. Tokio, vol I; 1970. p. 11.

183. Gil-Vernet JM. New surgical concepts in remooving renal calculi. Urol Int. 1965;20:225–88.

184. Gil-Vernet IM. Intrasinusale surgery. In: Wickham JEA, editor. Intrarenal surgery. Edinburgh, London, Melbourne, New York: Churchill-Livingstone; 1984. p. 129–48.

185. Rocca Rossetti S. Renstructive operations on intrarenal collecting system. In: Wickham JEA, editor. Intrarenal surgery. Edinburgh, London, Melbourne, New York: Churchill-Livingstone; 1984. p. 260–70.

186. Pagano S. L'Uretere, malattie e sintomi. Milano: Springer; 2010.
187. Acher PL, et al. Ureyeroscopic holmium laser endopyelotomy for uretrropyelic junction stenosis after pyeloplasty. J Endourol. 2009;23(6):899–902.
188. Milhina PM, et al. Primary endoscopic management versus open revision of ureteroenteric anastomosis strictures after urinary diversion. Single insitution contemporary series. J Endourol Marc. 2009;23(3):551–5.
189. Bach T, Geavlete B, Herrmann TW, Gross AJ. Retrograde blind endoureterotomy for subtotal ureteral strictures: a new technique. J Endourol. 2008;22(11):25–70.
190. Godor Y, Gabr AH, Faeber GJ, Roberts WH, Stuart Wolff J. Success of laser endoureterotomy of ureteral strictures associated with ureteral stones is related to stone impaction. J Endourol. 2008;22(11):2507–12.
191. Elkhader K, Houtani A, Nouri M, Ibn Attiya A, Hachini M, Rakrissa A. Une complication execionelle de l'endopyèlotomie : l'invagination urètèral (à propos d'un cas). Prog Urol. 1997; 273–6.
192. Martin X, Ndoye A, Konan PG, Feltosa Taja LC, Gelet A, Dawahra M, Dubernard M. Hazards of lumbar ureteroscpy: a Propos of 4 cases of avulsion of ureter. Prog Urol. 1998;8(3):358–62.
193. Rocca Rossetti S. Intrarenal plastic surgery for the collecting system. In: Proceedings international symposium. Wien: Ed. Porpacsy 133; 1979.
194. Culp D. Pyeloplastic thecnique. In: Flocks RH, Culp D, editors. Surgical urology, year book. 2nd ed. Chicago: Medical Publishers; 1963. p. 82.
195. Rocca Rossetti S. Reconstructive operations on the intrarenal collecting system. In: Wickham EA, editor. Intrarenal surgery. Edinburgh, London, Melbourne, New York: Churcill Liveingstone; 1984. p. 268.
196. Collins WE, Rege PR, Scott AC. Hamilton stewart nephroplasty. Can J Surg. 1867;10:53–9. in J.T. Grayhack: The Year Book of Urology, 1967–68
197. Smith PJ. Hamilton syewart nephroplasty. Proc R Soc Med. 1973;65(11):1021–3.
198. Smith PJ, Dunn M, Roberts JB. Nephroplasty in the management of hydronephrosis. Proc Urol Intern. 1979;51(14):245–8.

199. Hamilton Stewart HH. The nephroplasty procedure in the treatment of hydronephrosis. Br J Urol Int. 1957;23(3):277–86.
200. Wiu Z et al. Robotic versus open partial nephrectomy: a systematic and meta-analisis. Plos one. 2014;
201. Omar M, et al. Robotic versus open partial nephrectomy a systematic review and meta-analisis. Eur Urol. 2012;62(6):1023–33.
202. Ficarra V, Novara G, Volpe A, Motrie A. Robotic assisted versus traditional laparoscopic partial nephrectomy: time meta-analisis has not jet arrived. Br J Urol Int. 2013;112(4):E334–6.
203. Volpe A, et al. Perioperative and renal functional outcomes of elective robot. Assisted partial nephrectomy for renal tumors with high surgical complexity. Br J Urol Int. 2014;114(6):903–9.
204. Gill S, Eisenberg MS, et al. Zero ischemia partial nephrectomy: novel laparoscopic and robotic technique. Eur Urol. 2011;8(1):128–54.
205. Aron M, Koenig P, et al. Robotic and laparoscopic partial nephrectomy a matched-pair comparison from a high volume centre. Br J Urol Int. 2008;102(1):86–92.
206. Uberoi J, Disick GS, Munver R. Minimally invasive surgical management of pelvic-ureteric jonctionobstruction: update on the current status of robotic. Assisted pyeloplasty. Br J Urol Int. 2009;104(11):1721–9.
207. Muto G. Comunicazione personale. 2016.
208. Muto G. Comunicazione personale. 2016.
209. Porpiglia F. Comunicazione personale. 2016.
210. Basiri A, et al. Comparison of safety and efficacy of laparoscopic pyelolithotomy versus percutaneous nephrolithotomy in patients with renal pelvic stones: a randomized clinical trial. Urol J. 2014;11(6):1932–7.